2. Quinoa Salad with Chickpeas and Lemon Dressing

Ingredient:

- 1 cup uncooked quinoa, rinsed
- 1 (15 oz) can chickpeas, drained and rinsed
- 1 cup diced cucumber
- 1/2 cup diced red bell pepper
- 1/4 cup chopped fresh parsley
- 2 tbsp chopped fresh mint
- For the Dressing:
- 2 tbsp olive oil
- 2 tbsp lemon juice
- 1 tbsp Dijon mustard
- 1 garlic clove, minced
- 1 tsp honey
- Salt and pepper to taste

Instructions:

1. Cook the quinoa according to package instructions. Allow to cool.

2. In a large bowl, combine the cooked quinoa, chickpeas, cucumber, bell pepper, parsley, and mint.

3. In a small bowl, whisk together the olive oil, lemon juice, Dijon, garlic, and honey. Season with salt and pepper.

4. Pour the dressing over the quinoa salad and toss to coat evenly.

5. Serve chilled or at room temperature.

This quinoa salad is a great source of plant·based protein, fiber, and healthy fats. The chickpeas and quinoa provide a filling and satisfying base, while the fresh vegetables and herbs add crunch and flavor. The lemon dressing brightens up the whole dish. This salad can be enjoyed on its own or served as a side.

3. Grilled Salmon with Steamed Vegetables

Ingredient:

• 4 (6 oz) salmon fillets
• 2 tbsp olive oil
• Salt and pepper to taste
• 1 cup broccoli florets
• 1 cup sliced zucchini
• 1 cup sliced carrots
• 1/4 cup water

Instructions:

1. Preheat grill or grill pan to medium•high heat.

2. Brush the salmon fillets with olive oil and season with salt and pepper.

3. Grill the salmon for 4•6 minutes per side, or until it flakes easily with a fork.

4. While the salmon is grilling, place the broccoli, zucchini, and carrots in a steamer basket. Steam for 5•7 minutes, until vegetables are tender•crisp.

5. Remove the steamed vegetables from the heat and transfer to a serving bowl. Drizzle with a bit of the steaming liquid.

6. Serve the grilled salmon fillets immediately, alongside the steamed vegetables.

This meal is a great source of lean protein from the salmon, as well as fiber, vitamins, and minerals from the steamed vegetables. The combination of grilled salmon and steamed veggies makes for a healthy, balanced, and delicious dinner. The simple preparation allows the natural flavors to shine.

Welcome to the ***"Healthy Gut Flat Stomach Cookbook: 100+ Nutritious Recipes to Support Gut Health and Achieve a Flat Stomach."*** This cookbook is your comprehensive guide to enhancing digestive wellness and achieving a toned, flat stomach through the power of wholesome and nourishing recipes.

The Importance of Gut Health

A healthy gut is essential for overall well-being, influencing digestion, immunity, metabolism, and even mental health. When your gut is balanced and thriving, you experience better digestion, reduced bloating, increased nutrient absorption, and improved energy levels. The recipes in this cookbook are specifically crafted to support and nurture your gut health, helping you to feel your best from the inside out.

Nourishing Your Body, Supporting Your Goals

Beyond digestive health, this cookbook is designed to help you achieve a flat stomach. By focusing on ingredients that promote satiety, boost metabolism, and reduce inflammation, these recipes support your efforts to maintain a healthy weight and achieve a toned midsection. Each recipe is thoughtfully created to balance nutrition and flavor, ensuring that you enjoy delicious meals while working towards your health and fitness goals.

What You'll Find Inside

- ***100+ Nutritious Recipes:*** Explore a diverse collection of recipes that span from hearty breakfasts and satisfying lunches to flavorful dinners and guilt-free desserts, all designed to nourish your gut and support your quest for a flat stomach.

- ***Ingredient Insights:*** Learn about key ingredients that play a crucial role in promoting gut health and aiding in weight management, empowering you to make informed choices about your diet.

- ***Practical Tips:*** Discover practical tips on meal planning, prepping ingredients, and incorporating gut-friendly foods into your everyday meals, making healthy eating a seamless part of your lifestyle.

- ***Holistic Approach:*** Embrace a holistic approach to wellness that focuses not only on what you eat but also on how it supports your body's natural balance and vitality.

Your Journey to Wellness Starts Here

Whether you're looking to improve digestion, reduce belly fat, or simply nourish your body with wholesome ingredients, the "Healthy Gut Flat Stomach Cookbook" is your ultimate companion. Each recipe is crafted with care to ensure that you not only enjoy delicious meals but also support your journey towards optimal gut health and a flatter stomach.

Embrace the Benefits

Prepare to embark on a culinary adventure that will transform how you eat and feel. By nourishing your gut and supporting your health goals with these nutritious recipes, you're taking a proactive step towards a healthier, more vibrant life. Get ready to savor the flavors of good health and discover the joy of eating well for your gut and your waistline.

Here's to your digestive wellness and achieving your flat stomach goals with every meal!

1. Greek Yogurt Parfait with Berries and Granola

Ingredient:

- 1 cup plain Greek yogurt
- 1/2 cup fresh berries (such as blueberries, raspberries, or strawberries)
- 1/4 cup granola

Instructions:
1. In a parfait glass or small bowl, layer the Greek yogurt, berries, and granola, repeating the layers until you reach the top.

2. Serve chilled and enjoy!

This parfait is a great healthy snack or breakfast option. The Greek yogurt provides protein and probiotics to support gut health, while the berries are packed with antioxidants and fiber. The granola adds a crunchy texture and complex carbohydrates. Together, this parfait can be a satisfying and nutritious choice that may contribute to a flat stomach when enjoyed as part of an overall healthy diet and lifestyle.

4. Mixed Berry Smoothie with Spinach

Ingredient:

- 1 cup frozen mixed berries (such as blueberries, raspberries, and blackberries)
- 1 cup fresh spinach leaves
- 1 cup unsweetened almond milk
- 1/2 cup plain Greek yogurt
- 1 tbsp honey (optional)
- 1 tsp vanilla extract

Instructions:
1. Add all the ingredients to a high•powered blender.

2. Blend on high speed until smooth and creamy, about 1•2 minutes.

3. Taste and adjust sweetness with honey if desired.

4. Pour into a glass and enjoy immediately.

This smoothie is packed with nutrients from the mixed berries and spinach. The berries provide antioxidants, fiber, and natural sweetness, while the spinach adds a boost of vitamins, minerals, and phytonutrients. The Greek yogurt contributes protein and probiotics for gut health.

The almond milk and optional honey help create a creamy, smooth texture. This smoothie makes a great breakfast, snack, or post•workout recovery drink. The vibrant color and delicious flavor make it a healthy and satisfying choice.

5. Lentil Soup with Turmeric and Ginger

Ingredient:

- 1 cup dry brown or green lentils, rinsed
- 4 cups low•sodium vegetable or chicken broth
- 1 tbsp olive oil
- 1 onion, diced
- 3 garlic cloves, minced
- 1 tbsp grated fresh ginger
- 1 tsp ground turmeric
- 1 tsp ground cumin
- 1/4 tsp cayenne pepper (optional)
- Salt and pepper to taste
- Chopped fresh parsley for garnish

Instructions:

1. In a large pot, combine the lentils and broth. Bring to a boil over high heat.

2. Reduce heat to medium•low, cover and simmer for 20•25 minutes, until lentils are tender.

3. In a skillet, heat the olive oil over medium heat. Add the onion and sauté for 5 minutes until translucent.

4. Add the garlic, ginger, turmeric, cumin, and cayenne (if using). Cook for 1 minute, stirring constantly, until fragrant.

5. Transfer the onion•spice mixture to the pot with the cooked lentils. Stir to combine.

6. Season with salt and pepper to taste.

7. Ladle the lentil soup into bowls and garnish with chopped parsley.

This lentil soup is a nourishing and flavorful dish. The lentils provide plant•based protein and fiber, while the turmeric and ginger add anti•inflammatory benefits. The aromatic spices create a comforting, savory flavor. Serve this soup with crusty bread or a fresh salad for a complete and satisfying meal.

6. Whole Grain Toast with Avocado and Poached Egg

Ingredient:

• 2 slices whole grain bread, toasted
• 1 ripe avocado, mashed
• 2 eggs
• 1 tbsp white vinegar
• Salt and pepper to taste
• Red pepper flakes (optional)

Instructions:

1. Bring a medium saucepan of water to a gentle simmer over medium heat. Add the white vinegar.

2. Crack the eggs one at a time into a small bowl, then gently slide them into the simmering water. Poach the eggs for 3•5 minutes, until the whites are set but the yolks are still runny.

3. Remove the poached eggs from the water using a slotted spoon and set aside.

4. Spread the mashed avocado evenly over the toasted whole grain bread slices.

5. Top each slice with a poached egg.

6. Season with salt, pepper, and red pepper flakes (if using).

This open•faced toast makes for a nutritious and satisfying breakfast or snack. The whole grain bread provides complex carbs and fiber, the avocado offers healthy fats, and the poached egg contributes protein and nutrients like choline. The combination of creamy avocado, runny egg yolk, and crunchy toast creates a delicious and texturally•interesting dish. Enjoy this as a quick and easy way to fuel your body.

7. Stir•fried Tofu with Broccoli and Brown Rice

Ingredient:

• 1 cup uncooked brown rice
• 1 block (14 oz) extra•firm tofu, cubed
• 2 tbsp low•sodium soy sauce or tamari
• 1 tbsp sesame oil
• 1 tbsp rice vinegar
• 1 tsp honey
• 2 cloves garlic, minced
• 1 tbsp grated fresh ginger
• 2 cups broccoli florets
• 2 tbsp vegetable or avocado oil
• Salt and pepper to taste
• Chopped green onions for garnish (optional)

Instructions:

1. Cook the brown rice according to package instructions.

2. In a small bowl, whisk together the soy sauce, sesame oil, rice vinegar, and honey. Set aside.

3. Heat the vegetable oil in a large skillet or wok over medium•high heat. Add the tofu cubes and stir•fry for 3•4 minutes until lightly browned on all sides. Transfer to a plate.

4. In the same skillet, add the garlic and ginger. Stir•fry for 1 minute until fragrant.

5. Add the broccoli florets and stir•fry for 3•4 minutes until tender•crisp.

6. Return the tofu to the skillet and pour in the soy sauce mixture. Toss everything together and cook for 2•3 minutes until heated through.

7. Serve the stir•fried tofu and broccoli over the cooked brown rice. Garnish with chopped green onions if desired.

This stir•fry is a nutritious and flavorful vegetarian meal. The tofu provides plant•based protein, while the broccoli and brown rice offer fiber, vitamins, and minerals. The savory•sweet sauce complements the dish perfectly. Enjoy this as a quick and easy weeknight dinner.

8. Chicken and Vegetable Stir•fry

Ingredient:

• 1 lb boneless, skinless chicken breasts, cut into 1•inch pieces
• 2 tbsp low•sodium soy sauce
• 1 tbsp rice vinegar
• 1 tsp sesame oil
• 1 tbsp vegetable or avocado oil
• 3 cloves garlic, minced
• 1 tbsp grated fresh ginger
• 1 red bell pepper, sliced
• 1 cup broccoli florets
• 1 cup snow peas or snap peas
• 1 cup sliced mushrooms
• 2 green onions, sliced
• Salt and pepper to taste
• Cooked brown rice, for serving

For the Sauce:
• 2 tbsp low•sodium soy sauce
• 1 tbsp rice vinegar
• 1 tsp honey
• 1 tsp cornstarch

Instructions:

1. In a small bowl, combine the 2 tbsp soy sauce, 1 tbsp rice vinegar, and 1 tsp sesame oil. Add the chicken and toss to coat. Let marinate for 15 minutes.

2. In a small bowl, whisk together the sauce ingredients (2 tbsp soy sauce, 1 tbsp rice vinegar, honey, and cornstarch). Set aside.

3. Heat the vegetable oil in a large skillet or wok over high heat. Add the garlic and ginger and stir•fry for 1 minute until fragrant.

4. Add the marinated chicken and stir•fry for 3•4 minutes until lightly browned.

5. Add the bell pepper, broccoli, snow peas, and mushrooms. Stir•fry for 3•4 minutes until vegetables are tender•crisp. Pour in the sauce and toss everything together until the sauce thickens, about 1•2 minutes.

6. Remove from heat and stir in the green onions. Season with salt and pepper to taste. Serve the chicken and vegetable stir•fry over cooked brown rice.

9. Baked Sweet Potato with Black Beans and Salsa

Ingredient:

- 4 medium sweet potatoes
- 1 (15 oz) can black beans, drained and rinsed
- 1 cup prepared salsa
- 1/4 cup crumbled feta cheese (optional)
- Chopped fresh cilantro for garnish (optional)

Instructions:

1. Preheat the oven to 400°F. Pierce the sweet potatoes several times with a fork.

2. Bake the sweet potatoes for 45•60 minutes, until fork•tender. Allow to cool slightly.

3. Slice each sweet potato in half lengthwise. Scoop out the flesh into a bowl, leaving a thin layer attached to the skin.

4. Mash the sweet potato flesh with a fork. Stir in the black beans and salsa until well combined.

5. Spoon the sweet potato•black bean mixture back into the potato skins.

6. Return the stuffed sweet potatoes to the oven and bake for an additional 10•15 minutes, until heated through.

7. Remove from oven and top with crumbled feta cheese, if desired.

8. Garnish with chopped fresh cilantro before serving.

This baked sweet potato is a nutritious and satisfying vegetarian meal. The sweet potato provides complex carbs, fiber, and vitamins, while the black beans add plant•based protein and fiber. The salsa adds a flavorful kick. The feta cheese and cilantro are optional toppings that can enhance the dish. Enjoy this as a main course or a hearty side.

10. Chia Seed Pudding with Almond Milk

Ingredient:

• 1/4 cup chia seeds
• 1 cup unsweetened almond milk
• 1 tbsp maple syrup (or honey)
• 1/2 tsp vanilla extract
• 1/4 tsp ground cinnamon
• Fresh berries, for serving (such as blueberries, raspberries, or sliced strawberries)

Instructions:

1. In a medium bowl, whisk together the chia seeds, almond milk, maple syrup, vanilla, and cinnamon until well combined.

2. Cover the bowl and refrigerate for at least 2 hours, or overnight, stirring occasionally, until the mixture has thickened to a pudding•like consistency.

3. Divide the chia seed pudding into serving bowls or jars.

4. Top each serving with fresh berries.

5. Serve chilled.

This chia seed pudding is a nutritious and delicious breakfast, snack, or dessert. Chia seeds are rich in fiber, protein, omega•3 fatty acids, and antioxidants, which can support gut health. The almond milk provides a creamy base, while the maple syrup and cinnamon add natural sweetness.

The fresh berries add color, texture, and additional nutrients like vitamin C and antioxidants. This pudding can be enjoyed on its own or as part of a balanced diet that may contribute to a flat stomach when combined with regular exercise and other healthy lifestyle habits.

11. Green Tea with Lemon and Honey

Ingredient:

- 1 cup hot water
- 1 green tea bag
- 1 tbsp fresh lemon juice
- 1 tsp honey (or to taste)

Instructions:

1. Bring 1 cup of water to a boil.

2. Place the green tea bag in a mug and pour the hot water over it. Allow the tea to steep for 3•5 minutes.

3. Remove the tea bag and stir in the fresh lemon juice and honey.

4. Enjoy the green tea hot, or allow it to cool slightly before drinking.

This green tea with lemon and honey is a simple yet refreshing beverage that offers several health benefits:

Green Tea:
- Rich in antioxidants and polyphenols that may support overall health
- Contains L•theanine, an amino acid that can promote relaxation

Lemon:
- Provides vitamin C and other beneficial plant compounds
- May help aid digestion and support a healthy immune system

Honey:
- A natural sweetener with antioxidant properties
- May have antimicrobial effects and soothe the throat

Together, this combination of green tea, lemon, and honey creates a flavorful and nourishing drink that can be enjoyed hot or iced. It may contribute to a flat stomach as part of an overall healthy lifestyle.

12. Spinach and Mushroom Omelette

Ingredient:

• 3 eggs
• 1 tbsp milk or water
• 1 tsp olive oil
• 1/2 cup sliced mushrooms
• 1 cup fresh spinach leaves
• 2 tbsp shredded cheddar cheese (optional)
• Salt and pepper to taste

Instructions:

1. In a small bowl, whisk together the eggs and milk/water. Season with a pinch of salt and pepper.

2. Heat the olive oil in a non•stick skillet over medium heat.

3. Add the sliced mushrooms and sauté for 2•3 minutes until softened.

4. Add the spinach leaves and cook for 1 minute, stirring, until the spinach is wilted.

5. Pour the egg mixture into the skillet. As the eggs start to set around the edges, use a spatula to gently push cooked egg towards the center, tilting the pan to allow uncooked egg to flow to the edges.

6. When the eggs are mostly set but still a bit runny on top, sprinkle the shredded cheese (if using) over half of the omelette.

7. Fold the cheese•topped half over the other half and slide the omelette onto a plate.

8. Serve the spinach and mushroom omelette immediately, garnished with extra black pepper if desired.

This omelette is a nutritious and delicious breakfast or brunch option. The spinach and mushrooms provide fiber, vitamins, and antioxidants, while the eggs offer high•quality protein. The cheese is optional but adds extra creaminess and flavor. Enjoy this as part of a balanced diet that may contribute to a flat stomach.

13. Turkey and Vegetable Skewers

Ingredient:

- 1 lb ground turkey
- 1 zucchini, cut into 1•inch pieces
- 1 red bell pepper, cut into 1•inch pieces
- 1 red onion, cut into 1•inch pieces
- 8•10 cherry tomatoes
- 2 tbsp olive oil
- 1 tsp dried oregano
- 1 tsp garlic powder
- Salt and pepper to taste
- Wooden or metal skewers

Instructions:

1. Preheat grill or grill pan to medium•high heat.

2. In a large bowl, combine the ground turkey, 1 tbsp olive oil, oregano, garlic powder, salt, and pepper. Mix well until fully incorporated.

3. Thread the turkey mixture onto the skewers, alternating with the zucchini, bell pepper, onion, and cherry tomatoes.

4. Brush the skewers with the remaining 1 tbsp of olive oil.

5. Grill the skewers for 12•15 minutes, turning occasionally, until the turkey is cooked through and the vegetables are tender.

6. Serve the turkey and vegetable skewers hot.

These skewers make for a healthy and flavorful meal or appetizer. The lean turkey provides protein, while the vegetables offer fiber, vitamins, and minerals. The combination supports gut health with the fiber and antioxidants. When enjoyed as part of an overall balanced diet and active lifestyle, this dish may contribute to a flat stomach.

The grilled preparation adds a nice char and brings out the natural sweetness of the vegetables. Feel free to adjust the vegetable selection based on your preferences. Serve over a bed of greens or with a side of quinoa or brown rice for a complete and satisfying meal.

14. Cucumber and Tomato Salad with Olive Oil and Vinegar

Ingredient:

• 2 medium cucumbers, sliced
• 2 cups cherry or grape tomatoes, halved
• 1/2 red onion, thinly sliced
• 2 tbsp olive oil
• 2 tbsp red wine vinegar
• 1 tbsp lemon juice
• 1 tsp dried oregano
• Salt and pepper to taste
• Chopped fresh parsley for garnish (optional)

Instructions:

1. In a large bowl, combine the sliced cucumbers, halved tomatoes, and sliced red onion.

2. In a small bowl, whisk together the olive oil, red wine vinegar, lemon juice, and dried oregano. Season with salt and pepper.

3. Pour the dressing over the cucumber and tomato mixture and toss gently to coat.

4. Cover and refrigerate for at least 30 minutes to allow the flavors to meld.

5. Just before serving, give the salad another gentle toss.

6. Transfer to a serving bowl and garnish with chopped fresh parsley, if desired.

This cucumber and tomato salad is a refreshing and nutritious side dish or light meal. The combination of crisp cucumbers, juicy tomatoes, and tangy onion is complemented by the simple olive oil and vinegar dressing.

The vegetables provide fiber, vitamins, and antioxidants that can support gut health. When enjoyed as part of an overall balanced diet and active lifestyle, this salad may contribute to a flat stomach. It's a great option for summer gatherings or as a healthy accompaniment to grilled proteins.

15. Baked Cod with Quinoa and Roasted Vegetables

Ingredient:

• 4 (6 oz) cod fillets
• 1 cup uncooked quinoa, rinsed
• 2 cups mixed vegetables (such as broccoli florets, diced sweet potato, and sliced zucchini)
• 2 tbsp olive oil, divided
• 1 tsp garlic powder
• 1 tsp paprika
• Salt and pepper to taste
• Lemon wedges for serving

Instructions:

1. Preheat the oven to 400°F. Line a baking sheet with parchment paper.

2. In a medium saucepan, cook the quinoa according to package instructions. Fluff with a fork and set aside.

3. Toss the mixed vegetables with 1 tbsp of the olive oil, garlic powder, paprika, salt, and pepper. Spread in a single layer on the prepared baking sheet.

4. Roast the vegetables for 15•20 minutes, until tender and lightly browned.

5. Meanwhile, place the cod fillets on a separate baking sheet. Brush the top of the cod with the remaining 1 tbsp of olive oil and season with salt and pepper.

6. Bake the cod for 12•15 minutes, until it flakes easily with a fork.

7. Serve the baked cod over the cooked quinoa, topped with the roasted vegetables. Garnish with lemon wedges.

This meal is a nutritious and well•balanced dish. The cod provides lean protein, while the quinoa and roasted vegetables offer complex carbs, fiber, and a variety of vitamins and minerals. The combination supports gut health and may contribute to a flat stomach when enjoyed as part of an overall healthy lifestyle.

The simple seasoning allows the natural flavors of the ingredients to shine. Feel free to adjust the vegetable selection based on your preferences.

16. Sautéed Spinach with Garlic

Ingredient:

• 1 lb fresh spinach, washed and stems removed
• 2 tbsp olive oil
• 3 cloves garlic, minced
• 1/4 tsp red pepper flakes (optional)
• Salt and pepper to taste

Instructions:

1. In a large skillet or wok, heat the olive oil over medium heat.

2. Add the minced garlic and red pepper flakes (if using) to the hot oil. Cook for 1 minute, stirring constantly, until fragrant.

3. Add the fresh spinach to the skillet in batches, if needed, and sauté for 2•3 minutes, stirring frequently, until the spinach is wilted and tender.

4. Season the sautéed spinach with salt and pepper to taste.

5. Serve the garlicky sautéed spinach warm, as a side dish.

This simple sautéed spinach dish is a quick and easy way to enjoy the nutritional benefits of this leafy green vegetable. Spinach is packed with vitamins, minerals, and antioxidants that can support overall health and gut health.

The garlic adds flavor and may also provide some health benefits, such as anti•inflammatory properties. The optional red pepper flakes provide a subtle heat that can complement the spinach nicely.

This sautéed spinach makes a great side dish to pair with lean proteins, whole grains, or other roasted vegetables. It's a versatile and nutrient•dense addition to a balanced diet that may contribute to a flat stomach when combined with regular exercise and other healthy lifestyle habits.

17. Oatmeal with Fresh Fruit and Nuts

Ingredient:

- 1 cup old•fashioned rolled oats
- 2 cups unsweetened almond milk (or milk of your choice)
- 1 tbsp honey (optional)
- 1/2 cup fresh berries (such as blueberries, raspberries, or sliced strawberries)
- 2 tbsp chopped walnuts or almonds
- Cinnamon to taste

Instructions:

1. In a medium saucepan, combine the rolled oats and almond milk. Bring to a simmer over medium heat, stirring occasionally.

2. Reduce heat to low and continue cooking the oatmeal for 5•7 minutes, stirring frequently, until thickened to your desired consistency.

3. Remove the oatmeal from heat and stir in the honey, if using.

4. Transfer the oatmeal to serving bowls.

5. Top each serving with fresh berries, chopped nuts, and a sprinkle of cinnamon.

This oatmeal dish is a nutritious and satisfying breakfast option. The rolled oats provide complex carbohydrates, fiber, and protein to help keep you feeling full and energized. The fresh fruit adds natural sweetness, vitamins, and antioxidants, while the nuts contribute healthy fats and additional fiber.

The combination of the whole grains, fiber, protein, and healthy fats in this oatmeal can support gut health and may contribute to a flat stomach when enjoyed as part of an overall balanced diet and active lifestyle.

Feel free to customize the toppings based on your preferences or what's in season. This oatmeal can be enjoyed warm or chilled, making it a versatile and nourishing breakfast choice.

18. Steamed Edamame

Ingredient:

• 1 lb fresh edamame in the pod
• 1 tsp coarse sea salt (or to taste)

Instructions:

1. Bring a large pot of water to a boil over high heat.

2. Add the edamame pods to the boiling water. Cover and steam for 5•7 minutes, until the pods are bright green and tender.

3. Drain the edamame and transfer to a serving bowl.

4. Sprinkle the steamed edamame with the coarse sea salt, to taste.

5. Serve the edamame warm, providing small bowls for guests to squeeze the edamame beans out of the pods and enjoy.

Edamame is a nutritious snack or appetizer made from immature soybeans. They are a good source of plant•based protein, fiber, vitamins, and minerals. The simple steaming process helps preserve the nutrients and natural flavors of the edamame.

The coarse sea salt adds a nice contrast to the slightly sweet and nutty taste of the edamame. This dish can be enjoyed as a healthy snack or side dish. The fiber and protein in edamame may contribute to feelings of fullness and support gut health as part of an overall balanced diet.

Steamed edamame is a versatile and easy•to•prepare option that can be a great addition to a diet that may help contribute to a flat stomach when combined with regular exercise and other healthy lifestyle habits.

19. Caprese Salad with Balsamic Glaze

Ingredient:

- 8 oz fresh mozzarella cheese, sliced
- 2 medium tomatoes, sliced
- 1/4 cup fresh basil leaves
- 2 tbsp extra•virgin olive oil
- 2 tbsp balsamic glaze
- Salt and pepper to taste

Instructions:

1. Arrange the sliced mozzarella and tomatoes on a serving platter or plate.

2. Scatter the fresh basil leaves over the top.

3. Drizzle the olive oil and balsamic glaze over the salad.

4. Season with salt and pepper to taste.

5. Serve immediately.

This Caprese salad is a classic Italian dish that showcases the fresh, vibrant flavors of ripe tomatoes, creamy mozzarella, and fragrant basil. The balsamic glaze adds a sweet and tangy element that complements the other ingredients perfectly.

Tomatoes are a great source of the antioxidant lycopene, while mozzarella provides protein and calcium. Basil is rich in vitamins and has anti•inflammatory properties. The olive oil contains healthy monounsaturated fats.

This simple salad makes a refreshing and nutritious side dish or light meal. It can be enjoyed as part of a balanced diet that may contribute to a flat stomach when combined with regular exercise and other healthy lifestyle habits.

Feel free to adjust the ingredient amounts based on your preferences. You can also try adding a balsamic reduction or balsamic vinegar instead of the glaze, if desired.

20. Shrimp and Vegetable Stir•fry

Ingredient:

• 1 lb large shrimp, peeled and deveined
• 2 tbsp low•sodium soy sauce
• 1 tbsp rice vinegar
• 1 tsp sesame oil
• 2 tbsp vegetable or avocado oil
• 3 cloves garlic, minced
• 1 tbsp grated fresh ginger
• 1 red bell pepper, sliced
• 1 cup broccoli florets

• 1 cup snow peas or snap peas
• 1 cup sliced mushrooms
• 2 green onions, sliced
• Salt and pepper to taste
• Cooked brown rice, for serving

For the Sauce:
• 2 tbsp low•sodium soy sauce
• 1 tbsp rice vinegar
• 1 tsp honey
• 1 tsp cornstarch

Instructions:

1. In a small bowl, combine the shrimp, 2 tbsp soy sauce, 1 tbsp rice vinegar, and 1 tsp sesame oil. Toss to coat and let marinate for 15 minutes.

2. In a small bowl, whisk together the sauce ingredients (2 tbsp soy sauce, 1 tbsp rice vinegar, honey, and cornstarch). Set aside.

3. Heat the vegetable oil in a large skillet or wok over high heat. Add the garlic and ginger and stir•fry for 1 minute until fragrant.

4. Add the marinated shrimp and stir•fry for 2•3 minutes until partially cooked.

5. Add the bell pepper, broccoli, snow peas, and mushrooms. Stir•fry for 3•4 minutes until the vegetables are tender•crisp.

6. Pour in the prepared sauce and toss everything together until the sauce thickens, about 1•2 minutes.

7. Remove from heat and stir in the green onions. Season with salt and pepper to taste. Serve the shrimp and vegetable stir•fry over cooked brown rice.

This shrimp and vegetable stir•fry is a quick, healthy, and flavorful meal. The shrimp provides lean protein, while the vegetables offer fiber, vitamins, and antioxidants. The savory sauce ties all the flavors together. Enjoy this as part of a balanced diet that may contribute to a flat stomach.

21. Grilled Chicken Caesar Salad

Ingredient:

- 2 boneless, skinless chicken breasts
- 2 tbsp olive oil, divided
- 1 tsp garlic powder
- Salt and pepper to taste
- 6 cups chopped romaine lettuce
- 1/2 cup shredded Parmesan cheese
- 1/4 cup Caesar salad dressing
- 1 cup croutons
- Lemon wedges for serving (optional)

Instructions:

1. Preheat grill or grill pan to medium·high heat.

2. Brush the chicken breasts with 1 tbsp of the olive oil and season with garlic powder, salt, and pepper.

3. Grill the chicken for 5·7 minutes per side, until cooked through. Allow to rest for 5 minutes, then slice or chop the chicken.

4. In a large salad bowl, combine the chopped romaine lettuce, grilled chicken, Parmesan cheese, and croutons.

5. Drizzle the remaining 1 tbsp of olive oil and the Caesar dressing over the salad. Toss gently to coat.

6. Serve the grilled chicken Caesar salad immediately, with lemon wedges on the side if desired.

This grilled chicken Caesar salad is a nutritious and satisfying main dish. The romaine lettuce provides fiber and vitamins, while the grilled chicken adds lean protein. The Parmesan cheese and Caesar dressing contribute creaminess and flavor.

The combination of greens, protein, and healthy fats from the olive oil and dressing can help support gut health and may contribute to a flat stomach when enjoyed as part of an overall balanced diet and active lifestyle.

Feel free to adjust the ingredient amounts based on your preferences or the number of servings needed. You can also customize the salad by adding other fresh vegetables or swapping the romaine for a different type of leafy green.

22. Apple and Almond Butter Sandwich on Whole Grain Bread

Ingredient:

- 2 slices whole grain bread
- 2 tbsp creamy almond butter
- 1 small apple, thinly sliced
- 1 tsp honey (optional)
- Cinnamon (optional)

Instructions:

1. Spread the almond butter evenly on one slice of the whole grain bread.

2. Arrange the apple slices in a single layer on top of the almond butter.

3. Drizzle the honey over the apple slices, if using.

4. Sprinkle a light dusting of cinnamon over the apples, if desired.

5. Top with the second slice of whole grain bread to create a sandwich. Cut the sandwich in half and serve.

This apple and almond butter sandwich is a nutritious and satisfying snack or light meal. The whole grain bread provides complex carbohydrates and fiber, while the almond butter offers healthy fats and protein to help keep you feeling full.

The crisp apple slices add natural sweetness, crunch, and additional fiber. The optional honey and cinnamon can enhance the flavors even further.

This sandwich is a great source of nutrients that may support gut health and contribute to a flat stomach when enjoyed as part of an overall balanced diet and active lifestyle. The combination of complex carbs, fiber, protein, and healthy fats can help promote feelings of fullness and stable blood sugar levels.

Feel free to adjust the amount of almond butter or apple to suit your preferences. You can also try using different nut butters or fruit if desired.

23. Miso Soup with Tofu and Seaweed

Ingredient:

- 4 cups low•sodium vegetable or chicken broth
- 2 tbsp white or yellow miso paste
- 1 block (14 oz) firm or extra•firm tofu, cubed
- 1 cup thinly sliced shiitake mushrooms
- 1/2 cup chopped green onions
- 2 tbsp dried wakame seaweed (or other dried seaweed)
- 1 tsp sesame oil (optional)
- Pinch of red pepper flakes (optional)

Instructions:

1. In a medium saucepan, bring the broth to a gentle simmer over medium heat.

2. In a small bowl, whisk together the miso paste with a few tablespoons of the hot broth until smooth. Pour the miso mixture back into the saucepan, stirring to combine.

3. Add the cubed tofu, sliced shiitake mushrooms, green onions, and dried wakame seaweed to the broth. Simmer for 3•5 minutes, until the seaweed has softened.

4. Remove the soup from heat and stir in the sesame oil, if using.

5. Ladle the miso soup into bowls and garnish with a pinch of red pepper flakes, if desired.

6. Serve hot.

This miso soup is a nourishing and flavorful dish. Miso paste provides probiotics that can support gut health, while the tofu offers plant•based protein. The shiitake mushrooms, green onions, and seaweed add additional vitamins, minerals, and antioxidants.

The combination of the savory miso broth, tender tofu, and umami•rich vegetables makes this soup a satisfying and comforting meal. When enjoyed as part of an overall balanced diet and active lifestyle, this miso soup may contribute to a flat stomach.

Feel free to adjust the amount of miso paste or add extra vegetables based on your preferences. This soup can be enjoyed as a light main course or as a side dish.

24. Berry and Spinach Salad with Walnuts

Ingredient:

• 5 oz baby spinach leaves
• 1 cup mixed berries (such as blueberries, raspberries, and sliced strawberries)
• 1/4 cup chopped walnuts
• 2 tbsp balsamic vinaigrette
• 1 tbsp crumbled feta cheese (optional)
• Salt and pepper to taste

Instructions:

1. In a large salad bowl, combine the baby spinach leaves, mixed berries, and chopped walnuts.

2. Drizzle the balsamic vinaigrette over the salad and toss gently to coat.

3. Sprinkle the crumbled feta cheese over the top, if using.

4. Season with salt and pepper to taste.

5. Serve the berry and spinach salad immediately.

This salad is a nutritious and flavorful option that can be enjoyed as a main dish or a side. The spinach provides a base of fiber, vitamins, and minerals, while the berries add natural sweetness, antioxidants, and additional fiber.

The walnuts contribute healthy fats, protein, and crunch. The balsamic vinaigrette dressing complements the other ingredients with its tangy and slightly sweet flavor profile.

The combination of greens, berries, nuts, and a light dressing makes this salad a great choice to support gut health and potentially contribute to a flat stomach when incorporated into an overall balanced diet and active lifestyle.

Feel free to adjust the amounts of each ingredient to suit your preferences. You can also try adding other toppings like grilled chicken or toasted seeds for extra protein and nutrients.

25. Sardines on Whole Grain Crackers

Ingredient:

• 1 (4 oz) can of sardines in olive oil or water, drained
• 4•6 whole grain crackers
• 1 tbsp lemon juice
• 1 tsp Dijon mustard (optional)
• Salt and pepper to taste
• Chopped parsley or chives for garnish (optional)

Instructions:

1. Drain the sardines and transfer them to a small bowl.

2. Mash the sardines with a fork until they are broken down into flaky pieces.

3. Stir in the lemon juice and Dijon mustard (if using) until well combined.

4. Season the sardine mixture with salt and pepper to taste.

5. Spread the sardine mixture evenly onto the whole grain crackers.

6. Garnish with chopped parsley or chives, if desired.

7. Serve the sardine•topped crackers immediately.

This simple snack or light meal provides a nutritious boost of omega•3 fatty acids, protein, and other essential nutrients from the sardines. The whole grain crackers offer complex carbohydrates and fiber.

The lemon juice and optional Dijon mustard add a bright, tangy flavor that complements the rich, savory sardines. This combination of healthy fats, protein, and fiber can help support gut health and may contribute to a flat stomach when enjoyed as part of an overall balanced diet and active lifestyle.

Feel free to adjust the amount of sardines or seasonings to suit your taste preferences. You can also try using different types of whole grain crackers or topping the sardines with sliced cucumber or tomato.

26. Roasted Brussels Sprouts with Balsamic Vinegar

Ingredient:

• 1 lb Brussels sprouts, trimmed and halved
• 2 tbsp olive oil
• 1 tbsp balsamic vinegar
• 1 tsp honey
• Salt and pepper to taste

Instructions:

1. Preheat the oven to 400°F. Line a baking sheet with parchment paper.

2. In a large bowl, toss the trimmed and halved Brussels sprouts with the olive oil, balsamic vinegar, and honey. Season with salt and pepper.

3. Spread the Brussels sprouts in a single layer on the prepared baking sheet.

4. Roast for 20•25 minutes, tossing halfway, until the Brussels sprouts are tender and lightly browned.

5. Remove the roasted Brussels sprouts from the oven and transfer to a serving dish.

6. Serve the Brussels sprouts warm, drizzled with any remaining balsamic•honey glaze from the baking sheet.

These roasted Brussels sprouts with balsamic vinegar make a delicious and nutritious side dish. Brussels sprouts are high in fiber, vitamins, and antioxidants that can support gut health.

The balsamic vinegar and honey create a sweet•tangy glaze that caramelizes on the Brussels sprouts during roasting, adding depth of flavor. The simple preparation allows the natural flavors of the vegetables to shine.

This dish can be enjoyed as part of a balanced diet that may contribute to a flat stomach when combined with regular exercise and other healthy lifestyle habits. The fiber and nutrients in the Brussels sprouts can help promote feelings of fullness and overall well•being.

Feel free to adjust the amount of balsamic vinegar or honey to suit your taste preferences. You can also try adding other seasonings, such as garlic or Parmesan cheese.

27. Zucchini Noodles with Pesto and Cherry Tomatoes

Ingredient:

• 3 medium zucchini, spiralized or julienned into noodles
• 1/2 cup basil pesto
• 1 cup cherry tomatoes, halved
• 2 tbsp toasted pine nuts
• 2 tbsp grated Parmesan cheese (optional)
• Salt and pepper to taste

Instructions:

1. In a large bowl, combine the spiralized or julienned zucchini noodles with the basil pesto. Toss to coat the noodles evenly.

2. Add the halved cherry tomatoes and toss gently to incorporate.

3. Top the zucchini noodle mixture with the toasted pine nuts and grated Parmesan cheese (if using).

4. Season with salt and pepper to taste.

5. Serve the zucchini noodles with pesto and tomatoes immediately.

This dish is a delicious and nutritious way to enjoy the flavors of pesto and fresh vegetables. The zucchini noodles provide a low•carb, fiber•rich base, while the basil pesto adds a burst of flavor.

The cherry tomatoes contribute juicy sweetness and additional vitamins, while the pine nuts provide a crunchy texture and healthy fats. The optional Parmesan cheese adds a creamy, savory element.

This zucchini noodle dish is a great option to support gut health and may contribute to a flat stomach when incorporated into an overall balanced diet and active lifestyle. The combination of fiber, healthy fats, and antioxidants can help promote feelings of fullness and overall well•being.

Feel free to customize the recipe by using a different type of pesto or adding other fresh vegetables. This dish can be enjoyed as a main course or a side.

28. Chicken and Quinoa Stuffed Bell Peppers

Ingredient:

• 4 bell peppers, halved lengthwise and seeds removed
• 1 cup cooked quinoa
• 1 cup cooked and shredded chicken
• 1/2 cup diced onion
• 1 clove garlic, minced
• 1 tsp dried oregano
• 1/4 cup grated Parmesan cheese
• Salt and pepper to taste
• Chopped fresh parsley for garnish (optional)

Instructions:

1. Preheat the oven to 375°F. Arrange the bell pepper halves in a baking dish or on a rimmed baking sheet.

2. In a medium bowl, combine the cooked quinoa, shredded chicken, diced onion, garlic, oregano, and Parmesan cheese. Season with salt and pepper.

3. Spoon the chicken and quinoa mixture evenly into the bell pepper halves.

4. Bake for 25•30 minutes, until the peppers are tender and the filling is hot.

5. Remove the stuffed peppers from the oven and garnish with chopped fresh parsley, if desired. Serve the chicken and quinoa stuffed bell peppers warm.

These stuffed bell peppers are a nutritious and satisfying meal. The bell peppers provide fiber, vitamins, and antioxidants, while the quinoa and chicken offer a balanced source of complex carbohydrates and protein.

The combination of ingredients supports gut health with the fiber, probiotics, and anti•inflammatory properties. When enjoyed as part of an overall balanced diet and active lifestyle, this dish may contribute to a flat stomach.

Feel free to adjust the filling ingredients based on your preferences, such as using different herbs or adding diced vegetables. This recipe can also be made with ground turkey or lean ground beef instead of chicken.

Serve the stuffed peppers as a main course or alongside a fresh salad for a complete and nourishing meal.

29. Smoothie Bowl with Acai, Banana, and Coconut

Ingredient:

- 1 packet frozen acai puree
- 1 ripe banana, frozen
- 1/2 cup unsweetened almond milk
- 1 tbsp chia seeds
- 1 tbsp shredded unsweetened coconut
- 1 tbsp sliced almonds
- 1 tsp honey (optional)

Instructions:

1. In a high•powered blender, combine the frozen acai puree, frozen banana, and almond milk. Blend until smooth and creamy.

2. Pour the acai•banana smoothie base into a bowl.

3. Top the smoothie with the chia seeds, shredded coconut, sliced almonds, and a drizzle of honey (if using).

4. Serve the acai smoothie bowl immediately.

This smoothie bowl is a nutrient•dense and satisfying breakfast or snack option. The acai puree provides antioxidants, while the banana adds natural sweetness, fiber, and potassium. The almond milk creates a creamy texture.

The chia seeds are a great source of fiber, protein, and omega•3 fatty acids that can support gut health. The shredded coconut and sliced almonds provide healthy fats and a crunchy topping.

When enjoyed as part of an overall balanced diet and active lifestyle, this acai smoothie bowl may contribute to a flat stomach due to the combination of fiber, protein, and healthy fats that can help promote feelings of fullness and stable blood sugar levels.

Feel free to customize the toppings with other fresh fruit, nuts, seeds, or a drizzle of nut butter. This smoothie bowl is a versatile and nourishing way to start your day.

30. Baked Halibut with Asparagus

Ingredient:

- 4 (6 oz) halibut fillets
- 1 lb asparagus, trimmed
- 2 tbsp olive oil, divided
- 1 tsp lemon zest
- 1 tbsp lemon juice
- 2 cloves garlic, minced
- 1 tsp dried dill
- Salt and pepper to taste

Instructions:

1. Preheat the oven to 400°F. Line a baking sheet with parchment paper.

2. Place the halibut fillets on one side of the prepared baking sheet. Toss the asparagus with 1 tbsp of the olive oil and arrange on the other side of the baking sheet.

3. In a small bowl, combine the remaining 1 tbsp olive oil, lemon zest, lemon juice, garlic, and dried dill. Season with salt and pepper.

4. Drizzle the lemon•garlic mixture over the halibut fillets, making sure to coat them evenly.

5. Bake for 12•15 minutes, until the halibut is opaque and flakes easily with a fork, and the asparagus is tender•crisp. Serve the baked halibut immediately, with the roasted asparagus on the side.

This baked halibut and asparagus dish is a nutritious and flavorful meal. Halibut is a lean, high•protein fish that provides omega•3 fatty acids, which can support gut health. The asparagus is a great source of fiber, vitamins, and antioxidants.

The lemon•garlic seasoning adds a bright, savory flavor to the dish. When enjoyed as part of an overall balanced diet and active lifestyle, this meal may contribute to a flat stomach due to the combination of lean protein, fiber, and healthy fats.

Feel free to adjust the cooking time based on the thickness of your halibut fillets. You can also try different herbs or spices to season the fish and vegetables.

This baked halibut and asparagus makes a quick and easy weeknight dinner that supports overall health and well•being.

31. Cabbage and Apple Slaw with Yogurt Dressing

Ingredient:

- 4 cups shredded green cabbage
- 1 cup shredded red cabbage
- 1 apple, julienned or grated
- 1/4 cup plain Greek yogurt
- 2 tbsp apple cider vinegar
- 1 tbsp honey
- 1 tsp Dijon mustard
- Salt and pepper to taste
- Chopped fresh parsley for garnish (optional)

Instructions:

1. In a large bowl, combine the shredded green cabbage, shredded red cabbage, and julienned or grated apple.

2. In a small bowl, whisk together the Greek yogurt, apple cider vinegar, honey, and Dijon mustard. Season with salt and pepper.

3. Pour the yogurt dressing over the cabbage and apple mixture and toss to coat evenly.

4. Cover and refrigerate the slaw for at least 30 minutes to allow the flavors to meld. Just before serving, give the slaw another gentle toss.

6. Transfer the cabbage and apple slaw to a serving bowl and garnish with chopped fresh parsley, if desired.

This cabbage and apple slaw is a refreshing and nutritious side dish or light meal. The combination of green and red cabbage provides a variety of vitamins, minerals, and antioxidants. The apple adds natural sweetness and crunch.

The yogurt·based dressing is tangy, creamy, and lightly sweetened, complementing the other ingredients. The probiotics in the Greek yogurt can support gut health.

When enjoyed as part of an overall balanced diet and active lifestyle, this slaw may contribute to a flat stomach due to the fiber, protein, and healthy fats that can help promote feelings of fullness and stable blood sugar levels.

Feel free to adjust the ratio of green to red cabbage or try using different types of apples based on your preferences. This slaw can be served chilled or at room temperature.

32. Veggie Burger on Whole Wheat Bun

Ingredient:

• 1 15oz can black beans, drained and rinsed
• 1 cup cooked brown rice
• 1/2 cup rolled oats
• 1/4 cup breadcrumbs
• 1 egg, lightly beaten
• 1 tsp garlic powder
• 1 tsp onion powder
• 1 tsp cumin
• 1/2 tsp smoked paprika
• Salt and pepper to taste
• 4 whole wheat burger buns

Instructions:

1. In a large bowl, mash the black beans with a fork or potato masher until slightly chunky.

2. Add the cooked brown rice, rolled oats, breadcrumbs, egg, garlic powder, onion powder, cumin, smoked paprika, salt and pepper. Mix well until fully combined.

3. Divide the mixture into 4 equal portions and form into patties, about 1/2 inch thick.

4. Heat a large skillet over medium heat and add a bit of oil. Cook the veggie patties for 3•4 minutes per side, until lightly browned.

5. Serve the veggie burgers on the whole wheat buns. Top with your favorite condiments like lettuce, tomato, avocado, etc.

Enjoy your delicious and nutritious veggie burger on a whole wheat bun!

33. Hummus and Veggie Wrap

Ingredient:

- 4 whole wheat tortillas or wraps
- 1 cup hummus
- 1 cup shredded carrots
- 1 cup sliced cucumber
- 1 cup baby spinach or arugula
- 1/2 cup sliced red bell pepper
- 1/4 cup crumbled feta cheese (optional)
- Salt and pepper to taste

Instructions:

1. Spread about 1/4 cup of hummus evenly onto each whole wheat tortilla or wrap.

2. Layer the shredded carrots, sliced cucumber, baby spinach/arugula, and sliced red bell pepper on top of the hummus.

3. Sprinkle the crumbled feta cheese over the veggies, if using.

4. Season with a pinch of salt and pepper.

5. Fold the bottom of the wrap up, then fold in the sides and roll up tightly to enclose the filling.

6. Slice the wrap in half diagonally, if desired.

Serve the hummus and veggie wraps immediately or wrap them tightly in foil or parchment paper to enjoy later.

The combination of creamy hummus, crunchy veggies, and tangy feta makes this a delicious and nutritious vegetarian wrap. Enjoy!

34. Broccoli and Cauliflower Salad with Lemon Tahini Dressing

Ingredient:

Salad:
- 2 cups broccoli florets
- 2 cups cauliflower florets
- 1/2 cup sliced red onion
- 1/2 cup toasted slivered almonds
- 2 tablespoons dried cranberries

Lemon Tahini Dressing:
- 1/4 cup tahini
- 2 tablespoons lemon juice
- 1 tablespoon olive oil
- 1 garlic clove, minced
- 2•3 tablespoons water, to thin
- Salt and pepper to taste

Instructions:

1. In a large bowl, combine the broccoli florets, cauliflower florets, sliced red onion, toasted slivered almonds, and dried cranberries. Set aside.

Lemon Tahini Dressing:

1. In a small bowl, whisk together the tahini, lemon juice, olive oil, and minced garlic.

2. Add 2•3 tablespoons of water, one tablespoon at a time, until the dressing reaches your desired consistency. It should be pourable but still thick.

3. Season with salt and pepper to taste.

Assembly:

1. Pour the lemon tahini dressing over the broccoli and cauliflower salad and toss gently to coat.

2. Refrigerate for at least 30 minutes to allow the flavors to meld.

3. Serve chilled or at room temperature.

The creamy lemon tahini dressing complements the crunchy broccoli, cauliflower, and toasted almonds perfectly. This salad makes a great side dish or light main course.

35. Tuna Salad with Avocado and Greens

Ingredient:

- 2 (5 oz) cans of tuna, drained
- 1 ripe avocado, diced
- 1/4 cup diced celery
- 2 tablespoons diced red onion
- 2 tablespoons plain Greek yogurt
- 1 tablespoon lemon juice
- 1 teaspoon Dijon mustard
- Salt and pepper to taste
- 4 cups mixed greens (such as spinach, arugula, or kale)

Instructions:

1. In a medium bowl, gently mix together the drained tuna, diced avocado, celery, and red onion.

2. In a small bowl, whisk together the Greek yogurt, lemon juice, and Dijon mustard. Season with salt and pepper.

3. Pour the yogurt dressing over the tuna and avocado mixture and stir gently to combine.

4. Divide the mixed greens evenly among 2·3 plates or bowls.

5. Top the greens with the tuna salad mixture, distributing it evenly.

6. Serve immediately.

The creamy avocado and tangy yogurt dressing complement the flaky tuna perfectly. The greens add a nice crunch and freshness to the salad. This makes a delicious and nutritious lunch or light dinner.

36. Whole Grain Pasta
with Marinara Sauce and Spinach

Ingredient:

• 8 oz whole grain pasta (such as penne, fusilli, or spaghetti)
• 1 tablespoon olive oil
• 3 garlic cloves, minced
• 1 (28 oz) can crushed tomatoes
• 1 teaspoon dried oregano
• 1/4 teaspoon red pepper flakes (optional)
• Salt and pepper to taste
• 4 cups fresh spinach, roughly chopped
• 1/4 cup grated Parmesan cheese (optional)

Instructions:

1. Bring a large pot of salted water to a boil. Cook the whole grain pasta according to package instructions until al dente. Drain and set aside.

2. In a large skillet, heat the olive oil over medium heat. Add the minced garlic and cook for 1 minute, until fragrant.

3. Pour in the crushed tomatoes and stir in the dried oregano and red pepper flakes (if using). Season with salt and pepper to taste.

4. Bring the marinara sauce to a simmer and let it cook for 5•7 minutes, stirring occasionally, to allow the flavors to meld.

5. Add the cooked whole grain pasta and the chopped spinach to the skillet with the marinara sauce. Toss everything together until the spinach is wilted, about 2•3 minutes.

6. Remove from heat and serve immediately, garnished with grated Parmesan cheese if desired.

The whole grain pasta provides complex carbs and fiber, while the spinach adds a nutritional boost of vitamins and minerals. The simple marinara sauce ties it all together for a delicious and wholesome pasta dish.

Enjoy!

37. Roasted Beet and Goat Cheese Salad

Ingredient:

- 3-4 medium beets, peeled and cut into 1-inch cubes
- 2 tablespoons olive oil
- Salt and pepper to taste
- 5 oz mixed greens (such as spinach, arugula, or spring mix)
- 1/2 cup crumbled goat cheese
- 2 tablespoons toasted walnuts or pecans
- 2 tablespoons balsamic vinegar
- 1 tablespoon honey

Instructions:

1. Preheat your oven to 400°F (200°C).

2. Toss the cubed beets with the olive oil and season with salt and pepper. Spread them out in a single layer on a baking sheet.

3. Roast the beets for 25-30 minutes, stirring halfway, until they are tender and lightly caramelized. Allow to cool slightly.

4. In a large salad bowl, combine the mixed greens, roasted beets, crumbled goat cheese, and toasted nuts.

5. In a small bowl, whisk together the balsamic vinegar and honey to make the dressing.

6. Drizzle the balsamic honey dressing over the salad and toss gently to coat.

7. Serve the roasted beet and goat cheese salad immediately.

The earthy sweetness of the roasted beets pairs beautifully with the tangy goat cheese and the crunchy nuts. The balsamic honey dressing ties all the flavors together perfectly.

38. Baked Chicken with Sweet Potatoes

Ingredient:

• 4 boneless, skinless chicken breasts
• 2 medium sweet potatoes, peeled and cut into 1•inch cubes
• 2 tablespoons olive oil
• 1 teaspoon paprika
• 1 teaspoon garlic powder
• 1 teaspoon dried thyme
• Salt and pepper to taste
• 2 tablespoons chopped fresh parsley (optional)

Instructions:

1. Preheat your oven to 400°F (200°C).

2. In a large bowl, toss the cubed sweet potatoes with 1 tablespoon of the olive oil. Season with salt and pepper.

3. Spread the sweet potato cubes in a single layer on a baking sheet. Roast for 15 minutes.

4. While the sweet potatoes are roasting, place the chicken breasts in the same large bowl. Drizzle with the remaining 1 tablespoon of olive oil and season with paprika, garlic powder, dried thyme, salt, and pepper. Rub the seasoning all over the chicken.

5. After the sweet potatoes have roasted for 15 minutes, remove the baking sheet from the oven. Push the sweet potatoes to the sides of the sheet, creating a space in the middle. Place the seasoned chicken breasts in the center.

6. Return the baking sheet to the oven and continue baking for 25•30 minutes, or until the chicken is cooked through (internal temperature reaches 165°F/75°C) and the sweet potatoes are tender.

7. Remove the baking sheet from the oven and let the chicken and sweet potatoes rest for 5 minutes.

8. Serve the baked chicken and sweet potatoes warm, garnished with chopped fresh parsley if desired.

This simple one•pan meal is a great source of lean protein, complex carbs, and essential vitamins and minerals. Enjoy!

39. Steamed Mussels with Garlic and White Wine

Ingredient:

- 2 lbs (1 kg) fresh mussels, scrubbed and debearded
- 2 tablespoons olive oil
- 3 garlic cloves, minced
- 1 cup dry white wine
- 1/4 cup chopped fresh parsley
- 1 tablespoon unsalted butter
- Salt and freshly ground black pepper to taste
- Crusty bread, for serving (optional)

Instructions:

1. Rinse the mussels under cold running water, scrubbing off any dirt or debris. Remove the beards (the fibrous strings) by pulling them off with your fingers.

2. In a large pot or Dutch oven, heat the olive oil over medium heat. Add the minced garlic and cook for 1 minute, until fragrant.

3. Pour in the white wine and bring to a simmer. Add the mussels, cover the pot, and steam for 5•7 minutes, or until the mussels have opened up.

4. Using a slotted spoon, transfer the cooked mussels to a serving bowl, discarding any mussels that did not open.

5. Add the chopped parsley and butter to the pot with the cooking liquid. Stir until the butter has melted and the sauce is slightly thickened.

6. Pour the garlic•wine sauce over the mussels in the serving bowl. Season with salt and pepper to taste.

7. Serve the steamed mussels immediately, with crusty bread on the side for dipping in the flavorful broth (if desired).

Enjoy this simple yet elegant seafood dish! The combination of garlic, white wine, and parsley creates a delicious broth that complements the sweet, tender mussels.

40. Watermelon and Feta Salad with Mint

Ingredient:

• 4 cups cubed seedless watermelon
• 1 cup crumbled feta cheese
• 1/4 cup thinly sliced red onion
• 1/4 cup chopped fresh mint leaves
• 2 tablespoons balsamic glaze (or balsamic vinegar)
• 1 tablespoon olive oil
• Pinch of salt and freshly ground black pepper

Instructions:

1. In a large bowl, gently combine the cubed watermelon, crumbled feta cheese, sliced red onion, and chopped mint leaves.

2. Drizzle the balsamic glaze and olive oil over the salad. Gently toss to coat.

3. Season with a pinch of salt and freshly ground black pepper.

4. Serve the watermelon and feta salad immediately, or chill in the refrigerator for 30 minutes to allow the flavors to meld.

The sweet juicy watermelon pairs beautifully with the salty feta cheese, the peppery red onion, and the refreshing mint leaves. The balsamic glaze adds a touch of tangy sweetness to the salad.

This salad makes a great side dish or a light and refreshing summer main course. It's perfect for hot weather and can be enjoyed on its own or served with grilled meats or fish.

Enjoy this simple yet flavorful watermelon and feta salad!

41. Turkey Chili with Beans

Ingredient:

- 1 lb ground turkey
- 1 onion, diced
- 3 garlic cloves, minced
- 2 tablespoons chili powder
- 1 tablespoon ground cumin
- 1 teaspoon dried oregano
- 1/2 teaspoon smoked paprika
- 1/4 teaspoon cayenne pepper (optional, for heat)
- 1 (15 oz) can diced tomatoes
- 1 (15 oz) can kidney beans, drained and rinsed
- 1 (15 oz) can black beans, drained and rinsed
- 1 cup low•sodium chicken or vegetable broth
- Salt and pepper to taste
- Toppings: shredded cheese, diced avocado, chopped cilantro, sour cream

Instructions:

1. In a large pot or Dutch oven, cook the ground turkey over medium•high heat, breaking it up with a wooden spoon, until browned and cooked through, about 5•7 minutes. Drain any excess fat.

2. Add the diced onion and minced garlic to the pot. Cook for 2•3 minutes, until the onion is translucent.

3. Stir in the chili powder, cumin, oregano, smoked paprika, and cayenne (if using). Cook for 1 minute to toast the spices.

4. Pour in the diced tomatoes, kidney beans, black beans, and chicken/vegetable broth. Stir to combine.

5. Bring the chili to a simmer and let it cook for 20•25 minutes, stirring occasionally, until the flavors have melded and the chili has thickened.

6. Season with salt and pepper to taste. Serve the turkey chili hot, topped with shredded cheese, diced avocado, chopped cilantro, and a dollop of sour cream, if desired.

This hearty turkey chili is packed with protein, fiber, and bold Southwestern flavors. It's a comforting and satisfying meal, perfect for a chilly day.

42. Grilled Veggie Quesadilla with Guacamole

Ingredient:

Quesadilla:
• 8 whole wheat tortillas
• 1 cup shredded Monterey Jack or cheddar cheese
• 1 cup grilled or roasted vegetables (such as bell peppers, zucchini, onions, mushrooms)
• 2 tablespoons olive oil

Guacamole:
• 2 ripe avocados, pitted and mashed
• 1/4 cup diced tomato
• 2 tablespoons diced red onion
• 1 tablespoon chopped cilantro
• 1 tablespoon lime juice
• 1/2 teaspoon salt

Instructions:
1. Make the guacamole: In a medium bowl, mash the avocados. Stir in the diced tomato, red onion, cilantro, lime juice, and salt. Set aside.

2. Preheat a grill pan or outdoor grill to medium•high heat.

3. Lay 4 of the tortillas on a flat surface. Evenly distribute the shredded cheese and grilled/roasted vegetables over the tortillas.

4. Top each filled tortilla with another tortilla to create 4 quesadillas.

5. Brush the outside of the quesadillas lightly with olive oil.

6. Grill the quesadillas for 2•3 minutes per side, or until the cheese is melted and the tortillas are lightly charred.

7. Remove the grilled quesadillas from the heat and cut each one into 4 wedges.

8. Serve the grilled veggie quesadilla wedges warm, with the prepared guacamole on the side for dipping.

The combination of the grilled veggies, melted cheese, and creamy guacamole makes this a delicious and satisfying vegetarian meal. Enjoy!

43. Cauliflower Rice Stir•fry with Tofu

Ingredient:

• 1 head of cauliflower, riced (about 4 cups riced cauliflower)
• 1 block (14 oz) extra•firm tofu, cubed
• 2 tablespoons sesame oil
• 2 cloves garlic, minced
• 1 inch piece fresh ginger, grated
• 1 red bell pepper, sliced
• 1 cup sliced mushrooms
• 2 cups baby spinach
• 2 tablespoons low•sodium soy sauce or tamari
• 1 tablespoon rice vinegar
• 1 teaspoon sesame seeds (optional)
• Salt and pepper to taste

Instructions:

1. Prepare the cauliflower rice: Break the cauliflower into florets and pulse in a food processor until it resembles rice•sized granules. Set aside.

2. In a large skillet or wok, heat the sesame oil over medium•high heat. Add the cubed tofu and cook for 3•4 minutes per side, until lightly browned. Transfer the tofu to a plate and set aside.

3. In the same skillet, add the minced garlic and grated ginger. Cook for 1 minute, until fragrant.

4. Add the riced cauliflower, sliced bell pepper, and mushrooms to the skillet. Stir•fry for 5•7 minutes, until the vegetables are tender•crisp.

5. Stir in the cooked tofu, baby spinach, soy sauce, and rice vinegar. Cook for an additional 2•3 minutes, until the spinach is wilted.

6. Remove from heat and season with salt and pepper to taste.

7. Serve the cauliflower rice stir•fry warm, garnished with sesame seeds if desired.

This flavorful and nutritious cauliflower rice stir•fry is a great low•carb, vegetarian option. The tofu provides protein, while the vegetables and cauliflower rice make it a filling and satisfying meal.

44. Mango and Kale Smoothie

Ingredient:

- 1 cup frozen mango chunks
- 1 cup fresh kale, stems removed and leaves chopped
- 1 cup unsweetened almond milk (or milk of your choice)
- 1/2 banana, frozen
- 1 tablespoon honey (optional)
- 1 tablespoon chia seeds (optional)

Instructions:

1. Add the frozen mango chunks, chopped kale, almond milk, frozen banana, and honey (if using) to a high•powered blender.

2. Blend on high speed until the mixture is smooth and creamy, about 1•2 minutes.

3. If the smoothie is too thick, add a splash more almond milk and blend again until you reach your desired consistency.

4. Stir in the chia seeds (if using), reserving a few to sprinkle on top.

5. Pour the mango and kale smoothie into a glass and top with the remaining chia seeds.

6. Serve immediately.

The combination of sweet mango, nutrient•dense kale, and creamy almond milk makes this a delicious and healthy smoothie. The banana adds natural sweetness and creaminess, while the chia seeds provide a boost of fiber and omega•3s.

This smoothie is perfect for a quick breakfast, snack, or post•workout recovery drink. Adjust the amount of almond milk to reach your desired thickness.

Enjoy this refreshing and nutritious mango and kale smoothie!

45. Stuffed Portobello Mushrooms with Quinoa and Spinach

Ingredient:

- 4 large portobello mushroom caps, stems removed and chopped
- 1 cup cooked quinoa
- 1 cup fresh spinach, chopped
- 1/2 cup crumbled feta cheese
- 2 tablespoons olive oil
- 2 garlic cloves, minced
- 1/4 cup breadcrumbs
- Salt and pepper to taste

Instructions:

1. Preheat your oven to 400°F (200°C).

2. Gently clean the portobello mushroom caps with a damp paper towel. Remove the stems and chop them.

3. In a skillet, heat the olive oil over medium heat. Add the chopped mushroom stems and minced garlic. Sauté for 2·3 minutes until fragrant.

4. Add the chopped spinach to the skillet and cook for another 1·2 minutes until the spinach is wilted.

5. Transfer the spinach and mushroom mixture to a bowl. Stir in the cooked quinoa and crumbled feta cheese. Season with salt and pepper to taste.

6. Arrange the portobello mushroom caps, gill·side up, on a baking sheet. Spoon the quinoa and spinach mixture evenly into the mushroom caps.

7. Sprinkle the breadcrumbs over the top of the stuffed mushrooms.

8. Bake for 15·20 minutes, or until the mushrooms are tender and the filling is hot and lightly browned.

9. Serve the stuffed portobello mushrooms warm.

The earthy portobello mushrooms are the perfect vessel for the flavorful quinoa, spinach, and feta filling. This makes a delicious vegetarian main dish or side.

46. Greek Salad with Olives and Feta

Ingredient:

- 6 cups chopped romaine lettuce
- 1 cup cherry tomatoes, halved
- 1 cucumber, sliced
- 1/2 red onion, thinly sliced
- 1/2 cup pitted kalamata olives, halved
- 1/2 cup crumbled feta cheese
- 2 tablespoons olive oil
- 1 tablespoon red wine vinegar
- 1 teaspoon dried oregano
- 1/2 teaspoon Dijon mustard
- Salt and pepper to taste

Instructions:

1. In a large salad bowl, combine the chopped romaine lettuce, cherry tomatoes, sliced cucumber, thinly sliced red onion, and halved kalamata olives.

2. In a small bowl, whisk together the olive oil, red wine vinegar, Dijon mustard, and dried oregano. Season with salt and pepper to taste.

3. Drizzle the dressing over the salad and toss gently to coat.

4. Sprinkle the crumbled feta cheese over the top of the salad.

5. Serve the Greek salad immediately.

The crisp romaine lettuce, juicy tomatoes, crunchy cucumbers, and briny olives create a refreshing base for this salad. The tangy feta cheese and the simple vinaigrette dressing tie all the flavors together perfectly.

This Greek salad makes a great side dish or a light main course. It's packed with fresh, Mediterranean·inspired ingredients and is a healthy, delicious option.

47. Seared Scallops with Brown Rice and Peas

Ingredient:

- 1 lb sea scallops, patted dry
- 2 tablespoons olive oil
- 2 cups cooked brown rice
- 1 cup frozen peas, thawed
- 2 tablespoons lemon juice
- 2 tablespoons chopped fresh parsley
- Salt and pepper to taste

Instructions:

1. Heat a large skillet over high heat. Add the olive oil.

2. Season the scallops with salt and pepper. Working in batches if needed, sear the scallops for 2•3 minutes per side, until they are golden brown and cooked through. Transfer the seared scallops to a plate.

3. In the same skillet, add the cooked brown rice and thawed peas. Stir and cook for 2•3 minutes, until heated through.

4. Remove the skillet from heat and stir in the lemon juice and chopped parsley.

5. Divide the brown rice and pea mixture evenly among 4 plates or bowls.

6. Top each serving with 4•5 seared scallops.

7. Serve the seared scallops with brown rice and peas immediately, while the scallops are hot.

The seared scallops provide a delicate, sweet flavor that pairs beautifully with the nutty brown rice and fresh peas. The lemon juice and parsley add a bright, herbal note to the dish.

This is a simple yet elegant meal that's perfect for a weeknight dinner or a special occasion. Enjoy!

48. Chickpea and Spinach Curry

Ingredient:

• 2 tablespoons olive oil
• 1 onion, diced
• 3 garlic cloves, minced
• 1 tablespoon grated fresh ginger
• 2 teaspoons garam masala
• 1 teaspoon ground cumin
• 1 teaspoon ground coriander
• 1/4 teaspoon cayenne pepper (or to taste)
• 1 (15 oz) can chickpeas, drained and rinsed
• 1 (14 oz) can diced tomatoes
• 1 cup vegetable broth
• 4 cups fresh spinach, chopped
• 1/4 cup full•fat coconut milk
• Salt and pepper to taste
• Chopped cilantro for garnish (optional)

Instructions:

1. In a large skillet or pot, heat the olive oil over medium heat. Add the diced onion and cook for 5 minutes, until translucent.

2. Stir in the minced garlic and grated ginger. Cook for 1 minute, until fragrant.

3. Add the garam masala, cumin, coriander, and cayenne pepper. Stir to coat the onions and cook for 1 minute.

4. Pour in the drained and rinsed chickpeas, diced tomatoes, and vegetable broth. Bring the mixture to a simmer.

5. Reduce heat to medium•low and let the curry simmer for 10•15 minutes, stirring occasionally, until slightly thickened.

6. Stir in the chopped spinach and coconut milk. Cook for 2•3 minutes, until the spinach is wilted. Season with salt and pepper to taste.

7. Serve the chickpea and spinach curry over basmati rice or with naan bread. Garnish with chopped cilantro if desired.

This flavorful, vegetarian curry is packed with protein from the chickpeas and nutrients from the spinach. The blend of warm spices and creamy coconut milk creates a delicious, comforting dish.

49. Roasted Eggplant and Red Pepper Sandwich

Ingredient:

- 1 medium eggplant, sliced into 1/2•inch thick rounds
- 1 red bell pepper, sliced into strips
- 2 tablespoons olive oil
- Salt and pepper to taste
- 4 slices whole grain bread
- 2 ounces crumbled feta cheese
- 2 tablespoons pesto (store•bought or homemade)
- 2 cups baby spinach leaves

Instructions:

1. Preheat your oven to 400°F (200°C).

2. Arrange the eggplant slices and red pepper strips on a baking sheet. Drizzle with the olive oil and season with salt and pepper.

3. Roast the vegetables for 20•25 minutes, flipping halfway, until tender and lightly charred.

4. Remove the roasted vegetables from the oven and let them cool slightly.

5. To assemble the sandwiches, spread a thin layer of pesto on each slice of bread.

6. Layer the roasted eggplant and red pepper slices on two of the bread slices. Top with the crumbled feta cheese and baby spinach leaves.

7. Close the sandwiches with the remaining two bread slices.

8. Serve the roasted eggplant and red pepper sandwiches immediately.

The combination of the tender, flavorful roasted vegetables, tangy feta, and fresh spinach makes this a delicious and satisfying vegetarian sandwich. The pesto adds an extra burst of flavor.

You can serve this sandwich as is or pair it with a side salad or soup for a complete meal. Enjoy!

50. Coconut Milk Chia Seed Pudding

Ingredient:

• 1 (13.5 oz) can full•fat coconut milk
• 1/4 cup chia seeds
• 2 tablespoons maple syrup (or honey)
• 1 teaspoon vanilla extract
• 1/4 teaspoon ground cinnamon
• Pinch of salt
• Fresh fruit for topping (such as berries, mango, or kiwi)

Instructions:

1. In a medium bowl, whisk together the coconut milk, chia seeds, maple syrup, vanilla extract, cinnamon, and salt until well combined.

2. Cover the bowl and refrigerate for at least 4 hours, or overnight, stirring occasionally, until the chia seeds have thickened the mixture into a pudding•like consistency.

3. Once the chia seed pudding has set, give it a final stir to ensure it's evenly mixed.

4. Divide the coconut milk chia seed pudding into 4 serving bowls or jars.

5. Top each serving with your choice of fresh fruit, such as berries, mango, or kiwi.

6. Serve chilled and enjoy!

The combination of creamy coconut milk, nutrient•dense chia seeds, and sweet maple syrup creates a delicious and healthy pudding•like dessert or snack. The cinnamon adds a warm, comforting flavor.

This coconut milk chia seed pudding is perfect for meal prep, as it can be made in advance and stored in the refrigerator for up to 5 days. It's a great source of fiber, protein, and healthy fats.

Customize the toppings to your liking for a variety of flavors and textures. Enjoy this nourishing and satisfying chia seed pudding!

51. Shrimp and Avocado Salad

Ingredient:

- 1 lb cooked shrimp, peeled and deveined
- 2 ripe avocados, diced
- 1 cup cherry tomatoes, halved
- 1/2 red onion, thinly sliced
- 1/4 cup chopped fresh cilantro
- 2 tablespoons olive oil
- 2 tablespoons lime juice
- 1 teaspoon Dijon mustard
- Salt and pepper to taste

Instructions:

1. In a large bowl, gently combine the cooked shrimp, diced avocados, cherry tomatoes, sliced red onion, and chopped cilantro.

2. In a small bowl, whisk together the olive oil, lime juice, and Dijon mustard. Season the dressing with salt and pepper to taste.

3. Pour the dressing over the shrimp and avocado mixture and toss gently to coat.

4. Serve the shrimp and avocado salad immediately, or refrigerate for up to 30 minutes to allow the flavors to meld.

This refreshing and flavorful salad makes a great light lunch or dinner. The combination of tender shrimp, creamy avocado, juicy tomatoes, and tangy dressing is simply delicious.

You can serve the shrimp and avocado salad on a bed of mixed greens, or enjoy it on its own. It's also a great option for a summer potluck or barbecue.

Adjust the amounts of the ingredients to suit your taste preferences. Enjoy this healthy and satisfying shrimp and avocado salad!

52. Baked Falafel with Tahini Sauce

Ingredient:

Falafel:
• 1 (15 oz) can chickpeas, drained and rinsed
• 1/2 cup chopped parsley
• 1/4 cup chopped cilantro
• 2 garlic cloves, minced
• 1 teaspoon ground cumin
• 1 teaspoon ground coriander
• 1/2 teaspoon baking soda
• 1/4 teaspoon cayenne pepper
• 2 tablespoons all•purpose flour
• Salt and pepper to taste

Tahini Sauce:
• 1/2 cup tahini
• 1/4 cup water
• 2 tablespoons lemon juice
• 1 garlic clove, minced
• 1/4 teaspoon ground cumin
• Salt to taste

Instructions:

Falafel:

1. Preheat your oven to 400°F (200°C). Line a baking sheet with parchment paper.

2. In a food processor, combine the chickpeas, parsley, cilantro, garlic, cumin, coriander, baking soda, and cayenne. Pulse until the mixture is coarsely chopped but not pureed.

3. Transfer the falafel mixture to a bowl and stir in the flour. Season with salt and pepper.

4. Scoop the falafel mixture by the tablespoon and shape into small patties, about 1•inch thick.

5. Arrange the falafel patties on the prepared baking sheet.

6. Bake for 15•20 minutes, flipping halfway, until golden brown and crispy.

Tahini Sauce:

1. In a small bowl, whisk together the tahini, water, lemon juice, garlic, and cumin until smooth. Season with salt to taste.

Serve the baked falafel warm, drizzled with the tahini sauce. Enjoy!

The baked falafel is crispy on the outside and tender on the inside, while the creamy tahini sauce provides a delicious contrast. This is a healthier, oven•baked version of the classic Middle Eastern dish.

53. Spinach and Feta Stuffed Chicken Breast

Ingredient:

- 4 boneless, skinless chicken breasts
- 1 cup fresh spinach, chopped
- 1/2 cup crumbled feta cheese
- 2 tablespoons cream cheese, softened
- 1 garlic clove, minced
- 1 teaspoon dried oregano
- Salt and pepper to taste
- 1 tablespoon olive oil

Instructions:

1. Preheat your oven to 400°F (200°C).

2. In a medium bowl, mix together the chopped spinach, crumbled feta cheese, cream cheese, minced garlic, and dried oregano. Season with salt and pepper.

3. Using a sharp knife, cut a pocket into the side of each chicken breast, being careful not to cut all the way through.

4. Stuff the spinach and feta mixture evenly into the pockets of the chicken breasts.

5. Heat the olive oil in a large oven•safe skillet over medium•high heat.

6. Carefully place the stuffed chicken breasts in the hot skillet and sear for 2•3 minutes per side, until the outside is lightly browned.

7. Transfer the skillet to the preheated oven and bake for 20•25 minutes, or until the chicken is cooked through and the internal temperature reaches 165°F (75°C).

8. Remove the stuffed chicken breasts from the oven and let them rest for 5 minutes before serving.

Serve the spinach and feta stuffed chicken breasts warm. The melted cheese and spinach filling makes for a delicious and juicy chicken dish.

This recipe is easy to prepare and makes for a great weeknight dinner or impressive main course. Enjoy!

54. Brown Rice Sushi Rolls with Vegetables

Ingredient:

• 1 cup uncooked brown rice
• 2 cups water
• 1/4 cup rice vinegar
• 2 tablespoons sugar
• 1 teaspoon salt
• 1 cucumber, peeled, seeded and cut into thin strips
• 1 carrot, peeled and cut into thin strips
• 1 avocado, sliced
• 1 cup shredded purple cabbage
• 4•6 sheets of nori (seaweed sheets)

Equipment:
• Bamboo sushi mat

Instructions:

1. Cook the brown rice: In a medium saucepan, combine the brown rice and water. Bring to a boil, then reduce heat to low, cover and simmer for 30•35 minutes, until rice is tender. Fluff with a fork.

2. Make the sushi rice: In a small bowl, combine the rice vinegar, sugar, and salt. Pour this mixture over the cooked brown rice and stir gently to combine. Allow the rice to cool to room temperature.

3. Lay a sheet of nori on the bamboo sushi mat. Spread about 1/2 cup of the brown sushi rice evenly over the nori, leaving a 1•inch border at the top.

4. Arrange the cucumber, carrot, avocado, and purple cabbage in a line across the center of the rice.

5. Carefully lift the edge of the bamboo mat closest to you and roll it over the filling, pressing gently to secure the roll. Continue rolling the sushi, using the mat to shape it.

6. Wet the exposed nori border with a bit of water to help seal the roll. Repeat with the remaining nori sheets and fillings to make 4•6 sushi rolls. Use a sharp knife to slice each roll into 6•8 pieces.

55. Lentil and Vegetable Soup

Ingredient:

- 1 tablespoon olive oil
- 1 onion, diced
- 3 carrots, peeled and diced
- 3 celery stalks, diced
- 3 garlic cloves, minced
- 1 cup brown or green lentils, rinsed
- 6 cups low·sodium vegetable broth
- 1 (14.5 oz) can diced tomatoes
- 2 cups chopped kale or spinach
- 1 teaspoon dried thyme
- 1 bay leaf
- Salt and pepper to taste
- Chopped parsley for garnish (optional)

Instructions:

1. In a large pot or Dutch oven, heat the olive oil over medium heat. Add the diced onion, carrots, and celery. Cook for 5·7 minutes, stirring occasionally, until the vegetables are softened.

2. Stir in the minced garlic and cook for 1 minute, until fragrant.

3. Add the rinsed lentils, vegetable broth, diced tomatoes, kale/spinach, dried thyme, and bay leaf. Season with salt and pepper.

4. Bring the soup to a boil, then reduce the heat and let it simmer for 25·30 minutes, or until the lentils are tender.

5. Remove the bay leaf. Taste the soup and adjust seasoning as needed.

6. Serve the lentil and vegetable soup hot, garnished with chopped parsley if desired.

This hearty, nutritious soup is packed with fiber, protein, and vitamins from the lentils, vegetables, and greens. It's a comforting and satisfying meal, perfect for a chilly day.

Enjoy!

56. Grilled Steak with Roasted Vegetables

Ingredient:

Steak:
• 1 lb flank steak or skirt steak
• 2 tablespoons olive oil
• 2 teaspoons garlic powder
• 1 teaspoon onion powder
• Salt and pepper to taste

Roasted Vegetables:
• 2 cups cubed butternut squash
• 2 cups Brussels sprouts, halved
• 1 red bell pepper, cut into 1•inch pieces
• 1 red onion, cut into wedges
• 2 tablespoons olive oil
• 1 teaspoon dried thyme
• Salt and pepper to taste

Instructions:
1. Preheat your oven to 400°F (200°C).

Roasted Vegetables:
1. In a large baking sheet, toss the cubed butternut squash, Brussels sprouts, bell pepper, and red onion with the olive oil, dried thyme, salt, and pepper.
2. Roast the vegetables for 20•25 minutes, stirring halfway, until tender and lightly caramelized.

Steak:
1. Pat the steak dry with paper towels and season both sides generously with the garlic powder, onion powder, salt, and pepper.
2. Preheat a grill or grill pan to high heat.
3. Drizzle the steak with the olive oil and grill for 3•5 minutes per side, depending on thickness, for medium•rare doneness.
4. Transfer the grilled steak to a cutting board and let it rest for 5•10 minutes before slicing against the grain.

To Serve:
1. Arrange the grilled steak slices on a plate or platter.
2. Spoon the roasted vegetables around the steak.
3. Serve the grilled steak with roasted vegetables immediately.

57. Orange and Almond Salad with Citrus Dressing

Ingredient:

Salad:
• 5 oranges, peeled and segmented
• 1 cup baby arugula
• 1/2 cup sliced almonds, toasted
• 2 tablespoons crumbled feta cheese

Citrus Dressing:
• 2 tablespoons orange juice
• 1 tablespoon lemon juice
• 1 tablespoon olive oil
• 1 teaspoon honey
• 1/2 teaspoon Dijon mustard
• Salt and pepper to taste

Instructions:

1. Make the citrus dressing: In a small bowl, whisk together the orange juice, lemon juice, olive oil, honey, and Dijon mustard. Season with salt and pepper to taste.

2. In a large salad bowl, combine the orange segments, baby arugula, toasted sliced almonds, and crumbled feta cheese.

3. Drizzle the citrus dressing over the salad and gently toss to coat.

4. Serve the orange and almond salad immediately.

The sweet and juicy orange segments, peppery arugula, crunchy almonds, and tangy feta create a delightful flavor and texture combination in this salad.

The bright, citrusy dressing complements the other ingredients perfectly. You can adjust the amount of dressing to your preference.

This salad makes a refreshing and light meal on its own or can be served as a side dish. It's a great way to showcase the vibrant flavors of fresh oranges.

Enjoy this healthy and delicious orange and almond salad!

58. Baked Acorn Squash with Quinoa Stuffing

Ingredient:

- 2 acorn squash, halved and seeded
- 1 cup cooked quinoa
- 1/2 cup diced onion
- 1/2 cup diced celery
- 1/2 cup diced apple
- 1/4 cup chopped pecans
- 2 tablespoons dried cranberries
- 2 tablespoons chopped fresh parsley
- 1 tablespoon olive oil
- 1 teaspoon ground cinnamon
- Salt and pepper to taste

Instructions:

1. Preheat your oven to 400°F (200°C).

2. Place the acorn squash halves, cut•side up, on a baking sheet. Bake for 30•40 minutes, or until the squash is tender when pierced with a fork.

3. While the squash is baking, prepare the quinoa stuffing. In a medium skillet, heat the olive oil over medium heat. Add the diced onion and celery, and sauté for 5•7 minutes until softened.

4. Stir in the diced apple, chopped pecans, dried cranberries, and ground cinnamon. Cook for an additional 2•3 minutes.

5. Remove the skillet from heat and stir in the cooked quinoa and chopped parsley. Season the stuffing with salt and pepper to taste.

6. Once the squash is tender, remove it from the oven and carefully scoop out about 2•3 tablespoons of the flesh from each half, leaving a sturdy shell.

7. Add the scooped•out squash flesh to the quinoa stuffing mixture and stir to combine.

8. Spoon the quinoa stuffing back into the baked acorn squash halves.

9. Return the stuffed squash halves to the oven and bake for an additional 10•15 minutes, until the stuffing is heated through. Serve the baked acorn squash with quinoa stuffing warm.

59. Vietnamese Spring Rolls with Peanut Sauce

Ingredient:

Spring Rolls:
- 8 rice paper wrappers
- 1 cup shredded carrots
- 1 cup shredded cabbage
- 1 cup cooked vermicelli noodles
- 1/2 cup cooked shrimp, chopped (optional)
- 1/4 cup chopped fresh mint
- 1/4 cup chopped fresh cilantro

Peanut Sauce:
- 1/4 cup creamy peanut butter
- 2 tablespoons soy sauce
- 2 tablespoons rice vinegar
- 1 tablespoon honey
- 1 teaspoon sesame oil
- 1 garlic clove, minced
- 2•3 tablespoons warm water

Instructions:

Spring Rolls:

1. Fill a shallow dish with warm water. Dip one rice paper wrapper into the water for 10•15 seconds until softened.
2. Place the softened wrapper on a clean, damp surface. In the center, layer some shredded carrots, cabbage, vermicelli noodles, chopped shrimp (if using), mint, and cilantro.
3. Fold the bottom of the wrapper over the filling, then fold in the sides and roll up tightly to enclose the filling.
4. Repeat with the remaining wrappers and fillings.

Peanut Sauce:

1. In a small bowl, whisk together the peanut butter, soy sauce, rice vinegar, honey, sesame oil, and minced garlic.
2. Add 2•3 tablespoons of warm water and whisk until the sauce reaches your desired consistency.

To Serve:

1. Arrange the fresh spring rolls on a platter.
2. Serve the peanut sauce in a small bowl for dipping.

These light and refreshing Vietnamese spring rolls are packed with crunchy vegetables and optional shrimp. The creamy peanut sauce provides a delicious dipping accompaniment.

Enjoy these spring rolls as an appetizer or light main course. They're perfect for a warm weather meal.

60. Black Bean and Corn Salad

Ingredient:

• 1 (15 oz) can black beans, drained and rinsed
• 1 (15 oz) can corn, drained
• 1 red bell pepper, diced
• 1 cup cherry tomatoes, halved
• 1/2 red onion, diced
• 1/4 cup chopped fresh cilantro
• 2 tablespoons olive oil
• 2 tablespoons lime juice
• 1 teaspoon ground cumin
• 1/2 teaspoon chili powder
• Salt and pepper to taste

Instructions:

1. In a large bowl, combine the drained and rinsed black beans, drained corn, diced red bell pepper, halved cherry tomatoes, and diced red onion.

2. Add the chopped fresh cilantro to the bowl.

3. In a small bowl, whisk together the olive oil, lime juice, ground cumin, and chili powder. Season with salt and pepper to taste.

4. Pour the dressing over the black bean and corn salad and toss gently to coat.

5. Cover the salad and refrigerate for at least 30 minutes to allow the flavors to meld.

6. Serve the black bean and corn salad chilled or at room temperature.

This colorful and flavorful salad makes a great side dish or a light main course. The combination of black beans, corn, bell pepper, tomatoes, and onion provides a variety of textures and flavors.

The cumin and chili powder in the dressing give the salad a nice Southwestern flair. You can adjust the amounts of the spices to suit your taste preferences.

This black bean and corn salad is a perfect option for potlucks, barbecues, or as a healthy lunch or dinner. Enjoy!

61. Ratatouille

Ingredient:

• 2 tablespoons olive oil
• 1 eggplant, diced
• 1 zucchini, diced
• 1 yellow squash, diced
• 1 red bell pepper, diced
• 1 onion, diced
• 3 garlic cloves, minced
• 1 (14.5 oz) can diced tomatoes
• 2 tablespoons tomato paste
• 1 teaspoon dried thyme
• 1 teaspoon dried oregano
• Salt and pepper to taste
• Chopped fresh basil for garnish (optional)

Instructions:

1. In a large skillet or Dutch oven, heat the olive oil over medium heat.

2. Add the diced eggplant, zucchini, yellow squash, bell pepper, and onion. Cook, stirring occasionally, for 10•12 minutes, until the vegetables are starting to soften.

3. Stir in the minced garlic and cook for 1 minute, until fragrant.

4. Pour in the diced tomatoes and tomato paste. Add the dried thyme and oregano. Season with salt and pepper to taste.

5. Bring the mixture to a simmer, then reduce the heat to low. Cover and let the ratatouille simmer for 20•25 minutes, stirring occasionally, until the vegetables are very tender.

6. Taste and adjust seasoning as needed. Serve the ratatouille warm, garnished with chopped fresh basil if desired.

Ratatouille is a classic French vegetable stew that showcases the flavors of summer produce. The combination of eggplant, zucchini, squash, bell pepper, and tomatoes creates a delicious and satisfying dish.

This ratatouille can be served as a main course, side dish, or even as a topping for grilled meats or fish. It's a versatile and healthy option for any meal.

62. Poached Salmon with Dill and Lemon

Ingredient:

• 4 (6 oz) salmon fillets
• 4 cups water
• 2 tablespoons white wine vinegar
• 2 lemon slices
• 2 sprigs fresh dill, plus more for garnish
• Salt and pepper to taste

Lemon Dill Sauce:
• 1/2 cup plain Greek yogurt
• 2 tablespoons chopped fresh dill
• 1 tablespoon lemon juice
• 1 teaspoon Dijon mustard
• Salt and pepper to taste

Instructions:

1. In a large skillet or shallow saucepan, combine the water, white wine vinegar, lemon slices, and 2 sprigs of fresh dill. Bring the liquid to a gentle simmer over medium heat.

2. Carefully add the salmon fillets to the simmering liquid. Poach the salmon for 8•10 minutes, or until it flakes easily with a fork and reaches an internal temperature of 145°F (63°C).

3. Using a slotted spoon, transfer the poached salmon fillets to a plate.

Lemon Dill Sauce:
1. In a small bowl, whisk together the Greek yogurt, chopped fresh dill, lemon juice, and Dijon mustard. Season with salt and pepper to taste.

To Serve:
1. Place the poached salmon fillets on serving plates.
2. Drizzle the lemon dill sauce over the top of the salmon.
3. Garnish with additional fresh dill sprigs.
4. Serve the poached salmon warm.

The gentle poaching method keeps the salmon moist and tender, while the bright lemon and fragrant dill complement the fish perfectly. The creamy lemon dill sauce adds a delicious finishing touch.

63. Kale and Quinoa Salad with Lemon Vinaigrette

Ingredient:

- 1 cup uncooked quinoa, rinsed
- 2 cups chopped kale, stems removed
- 1 cup cherry tomatoes, halved
- 1/2 cup crumbled feta cheese
- 1/4 cup sliced almonds
- 2 tbsp olive oil
- 2 tbsp lemon juice
- 1 tsp Dijon mustard
- 1 tsp honey
- Salt and pepper to taste

Instructions:

1. Cook the quinoa according to package instructions. Allow to cool.

2. In a large bowl, combine the cooked quinoa, chopped kale, cherry tomatoes, feta cheese, and sliced almonds.

3. In a small bowl, whisk together the olive oil, lemon juice, Dijon mustard, and honey. Season with salt and pepper.

4. Pour the lemon vinaigrette over the salad and toss to coat evenly.

5. Serve immediately or refrigerate until ready to serve. The salad can be made a day in advance.

Enjoy your fresh and flavorful Kale and Quinoa Salad with Lemon Vinaigrette!

64. Tofu and Vegetable Stir•fry with Ginger Soy Sauce

Ingredient:

- 1 block (14 oz) extra•firm tofu, cubed
- 2 tbsp vegetable oil
- 2 cups mixed vegetables (such as broccoli, bell peppers, snap peas, carrots)
- 3 cloves garlic, minced
- 1 tbsp grated fresh ginger
- 3 tbsp low•sodium soy sauce
- 1 tbsp rice vinegar
- 1 tsp sesame oil
- 1 tsp honey
- Salt and pepper to taste
- Cooked rice, for serving

Ginger Soy Sauce:
- 3 tbsp low•sodium soy sauce
- 1 tbsp rice vinegar
- 1 tsp sesame oil
- 1 tsp honey
- 1 tsp grated fresh ginger

Instructions:

1. In a small bowl, whisk together all the ingredients for the ginger soy sauce. Set aside.

2. Heat the vegetable oil in a large skillet or wok over medium•high heat. Add the cubed tofu and cook, stirring occasionally, until lightly browned on all sides, about 5•7 minutes. Transfer the tofu to a plate.

3. Add the mixed vegetables to the skillet and stir•fry for 3•4 minutes until crisp•tender.

4. Add the garlic and ginger to the skillet and cook for 1 minute, until fragrant.

5. Return the tofu to the skillet and pour in the ginger soy sauce. Toss everything together and cook for 2•3 minutes, until the sauce has thickened slightly.

6. Serve the tofu and vegetable stir•fry immediately over cooked rice.

Enjoy your flavorful Tofu and Vegetable Stir•Fry with Ginger Soy Sauce!

65. Bell Pepper Nachos with Ground Turkey

Ingredient:

- 3 bell peppers, sliced into 1/4•inch thick rounds
- 1 lb ground turkey
- 1 packet taco seasoning
- 1 cup shredded cheddar cheese
- 1/2 cup diced tomatoes
- 1/4 cup sliced black olives
- 2 tbsp chopped fresh cilantro
- Sour cream, for serving (optional)
- Salsa, for serving (optional)

Instructions:

1. Preheat your oven to 400°F (200°C).

2. Arrange the bell pepper slices in a single layer on a large baking sheet.

3. In a skillet over medium heat, cook the ground turkey, breaking it up with a wooden spoon, until browned and cooked through, about 5•7 minutes. Drain any excess fat.

4. Sprinkle the taco seasoning over the cooked ground turkey and stir to coat evenly.

5. Spoon the seasoned ground turkey over the bell pepper slices, distributing it evenly.

6. Sprinkle the shredded cheddar cheese over the top.

7. Bake the nachos in the preheated oven for 10•12 minutes, or until the cheese is melted and bubbly.

8. Remove the nachos from the oven and top with the diced tomatoes, sliced black olives, and chopped fresh cilantro.

9. Serve the bell pepper nachos immediately, with sour cream and salsa on the side, if desired.

Enjoy your delicious and healthy Bell Pepper Nachos with Ground Turkey!

66. Edamame Hummus with Crudité

Ingredient:

Edamame Hummus:
• 1 cup shelled edamame, cooked and cooled
• 1/4 cup tahini
• 2 tbsp fresh lemon juice
• 2 cloves garlic, minced
• 1/4 cup olive oil
• 2 tbsp water
• 1/2 tsp ground cumin
• 1/4 tsp salt

Crudité:
• Assorted fresh vegetables (such as carrot sticks, cucumber slices, bell pepper strips, cherry tomatoes)

Instructions:

For the Edamame Hummus:
1. In a food processor, combine the cooked edamame, tahini, lemon juice, garlic, olive oil, water, cumin, and salt. Process until smooth and creamy, scraping down the sides as needed.
2. Transfer the hummus to a serving bowl.

For the Crudité:
1. Arrange the assorted fresh vegetables around the bowl of edamame hummus.

To Serve:
1. Serve the edamame hummus with the crudité vegetables for dipping.

Tips:
• You can adjust the amount of water to reach your desired consistency for the hummus.
• Feel free to use a variety of fresh vegetables, such as radishes, celery, and snap peas.
• For extra flavor, you can garnish the hummus with a drizzle of olive oil, a sprinkle of paprika, or chopped fresh herbs.

Enjoy your healthy and flavorful Edamame Hummus with Crudité!

67. Avocado and Chickpea Toast

Ingredient:

- 2 slices whole•grain bread
- 1 ripe avocado, mashed
- 1/2 cup cooked chickpeas, drained and rinsed
- 1 tbsp lemon juice
- 1 tsp olive oil
- 1/4 tsp ground cumin
- Salt and pepper to taste
- Chopped fresh cilantro or parsley for garnish (optional)

Instructions:

1. Toast the whole•grain bread until lightly golden brown.

2. In a medium bowl, mash the avocado with a fork or potato masher.

3. Add the cooked chickpeas, lemon juice, olive oil, and ground cumin. Stir to combine.

4. Season the avocado•chickpea mixture with salt and pepper to taste.

5. Spread the avocado•chickpea mixture evenly over the toasted bread slices.

6. Garnish the toasts with chopped fresh cilantro or parsley, if desired.

7. Serve the Avocado and Chickpea Toasts immediately.

Tips:
- For extra flavor, you can add a sprinkle of red pepper flakes or a drizzle of balsamic glaze.
- You can also top the toasts with sliced cherry tomatoes, crumbled feta, or a fried egg for a more substantial meal.
- This recipe can be easily doubled or tripled to serve more people.

Enjoy your delicious and nutritious Avocado and Chickpea Toast!

68. Grilled Swordfish with Mango Salsa

Ingredient:

Mango Salsa:
• 1 ripe mango, diced
• 1/2 red onion, finely chopped
• 1 jalapeño, seeded and finely chopped
• 1/4 cup chopped fresh cilantro
• 2 tbsp lime juice
• 1/4 tsp salt

Grilled Swordfish:
• 4 (6 oz) swordfish steaks
• 2 tbsp olive oil
• 1 tsp chili powder
• 1/2 tsp garlic powder
• 1/2 tsp salt
• 1/4 tsp black pepper

Instructions:

For the Mango Salsa:
1. In a medium bowl, combine the diced mango, chopped red onion, jalapeño, cilantro, lime juice, and salt. Stir to mix well. Cover and refrigerate until ready to serve.

For the Grilled Swordfish:
1. Preheat your grill to medium•high heat.

2. Pat the swordfish steaks dry with paper towels and brush both sides with the olive oil.

3. In a small bowl, mix together the chili powder, garlic powder, salt, and black pepper. Rub this seasoning mixture evenly over the swordfish steaks.

4. Grill the swordfish for 3•4 minutes per side, or until it flakes easily with a fork and is cooked through. Transfer the grilled swordfish steaks to a serving platter.

To Serve:
1. Top the grilled swordfish steaks with the prepared mango salsa.

2. Serve immediately, while the swordfish is hot.

Enjoy your delicious Grilled Swordfish with Mango Salsa!

69. Pear and Walnut Salad with Blue Cheese

Ingredient:

Salad:
• 5 oz mixed greens (such as spinach, arugula, and/or baby kale)
• 2 ripe pears, cored and sliced
• 1/2 cup crumbled blue cheese
• 1/2 cup toasted walnuts

***Dressing*:**
• 2 tbsp olive oil
• 1 tbsp balsamic vinegar
• 1 tsp Dijon mustard
• 1 tsp honey
• 1/4 tsp salt
• 1/8 tsp black pepper

Instructions:

1. In a large salad bowl, combine the mixed greens, sliced pears, crumbled blue cheese, and toasted walnuts.

For the Dressing:
1. In a small bowl, whisk together the olive oil, balsamic vinegar, Dijon mustard, honey, salt, and black pepper until well combined.

To Assemble:
1. Drizzle the dressing over the salad and toss gently to coat the greens and other ingredients evenly.

2. Serve the Pear and Walnut Salad with Blue Cheese immediately.

Tips:
• You can use any type of pear you prefer, such as Bartlett, Bosc, or Anjou.
• Toast the walnuts in a dry skillet over medium heat for 2•3 minutes, stirring frequently, until fragrant and lightly browned.
• For a heartier meal, you can add grilled chicken or shrimp to the salad.
• Adjust the amount of dressing to your liking, as some people prefer a lighter coating.

Enjoy your delicious and flavorful Pear and Walnut Salad with Blue Cheese!

70. Stuffed Bell Peppers with Turkey and Quinoa

Ingredient:

• 4 bell peppers (any color), halved lengthwise and seeds removed
• 1 lb ground turkey
• 1 cup cooked quinoa
• 1 small onion, finely chopped
• 2 cloves garlic, minced
• 1 tsp dried oregano
• 1 tsp ground cumin
• 1/2 tsp smoked paprika
• 1/4 tsp red pepper flakes (optional)
• 1 cup shredded cheddar cheese
• Salt and black pepper to taste

Instructions:

1. Preheat your oven to 375°F (190°C).

2. Arrange the bell pepper halves in a baking dish or on a rimmed baking sheet.

3. In a large skillet over medium heat, cook the ground turkey, breaking it up with a wooden spoon, until browned and cooked through, about 5•7 minutes. Drain any excess fat.

4. Add the chopped onion to the skillet and cook for 2•3 minutes, until softened. Stir in the minced garlic and cook for 1 minute more.

5. Remove the skillet from heat and stir in the cooked quinoa, dried oregano, ground cumin, smoked paprika, and red pepper flakes (if using). Season with salt and black pepper to taste.

6. Spoon the turkey and quinoa mixture evenly into the bell pepper halves, pressing it down gently.

7. Top each stuffed pepper with shredded cheddar cheese.

8. Bake the stuffed peppers in the preheated oven for 20•25 minutes, or until the peppers are tender and the cheese is melted and bubbly.

9. Serve the Stuffed Bell Peppers with Turkey and Quinoa warm.

71. Chicken and Spinach Stuffed Sweet Potatoes

Ingredient:

- 4 medium sweet potatoes, scrubbed clean
- 1 lb boneless, skinless chicken breasts
- 2 cups fresh spinach, chopped
- 1/2 cup shredded cheddar cheese
- 2 tbsp olive oil
- 1 tsp garlic powder
- 1 tsp onion powder
- Salt and black pepper to taste

Instructions:

1. Preheat your oven to 400°F (200°C).

2. Pierce the sweet potatoes several times with a fork. Place them directly on the oven rack and bake for 45•60 minutes, or until they are tender when pierced with a fork.

3. While the sweet potatoes are baking, season the chicken breasts with garlic powder, onion powder, salt, and black pepper.

4. Heat the olive oil in a skillet over medium•high heat. Add the seasoned chicken breasts and cook for 5•7 minutes per side, or until the chicken is cooked through and no longer pink in the center.

5. Remove the chicken from the skillet and let it rest for a few minutes. Then, shred or chop the chicken into bite•sized pieces.

6. Once the sweet potatoes are cooked, let them cool for a few minutes. Slice each potato in half lengthwise and scoop out the flesh, leaving a thin layer of sweet potato attached to the skin.

7. In a bowl, mash the scooped•out sweet potato flesh. Stir in the shredded chicken, chopped spinach, and shredded cheddar cheese. Season with additional salt and black pepper to taste.

8. Spoon the chicken and spinach mixture back into the sweet potato skins.

9. Return the stuffed sweet potatoes to the oven and bake for an additional 10•15 minutes, or until the cheese is melted and bubbly. Serve the Chicken and Spinach Stuffed Sweet Potatoes warm

72. Zucchini Noodles with Marinara Sauce

Ingredient:

• 4 medium zucchini, spiralized or julienned into noodles
• 2 tbsp olive oil
• 3 cloves garlic, minced
• 1 (28 oz) can crushed tomatoes
• 1 tsp dried oregano
• 1/2 tsp dried basil
• 1/4 tsp red pepper flakes (optional)
• Salt and black pepper to taste
• Grated Parmesan cheese for serving (optional)

Instructions:

1. Using a spiralizer or julienne peeler, cut the zucchini into long, thin noodles. Set aside.

2. In a large skillet, heat the olive oil over medium heat. Add the minced garlic and cook for 1•2 minutes, until fragrant.

3. Pour in the can of crushed tomatoes and stir in the dried oregano, dried basil, and red pepper flakes (if using). Season with salt and black pepper to taste.

4. Bring the marinara sauce to a simmer and let it cook for 5•7 minutes, stirring occasionally, to allow the flavors to meld.

5. Add the spiralized or julienned zucchini noodles to the skillet and toss them gently with the marinara sauce. Cook for 2•3 minutes, just until the zucchini noodles are tender but still have a bit of bite.

6. Remove the skillet from heat and serve the zucchini noodles with marinara sauce immediately.

7. Optionally, top with grated Parmesan cheese before serving.

Enjoy your healthy and delicious Zucchini Noodles with Marinara Sauce!

73. Broccoli and White Bean Soup

Ingredient:

- 2 tbsp olive oil
- 1 onion, diced
- 3 cloves garlic, minced
- 4 cups chopped broccoli florets
- 1 (15 oz) can white beans, drained and rinsed
- 4 cups low•sodium vegetable or chicken broth
- 1 tsp dried thyme
- 1/2 tsp salt
- 1/4 tsp black pepper
- Grated Parmesan cheese for serving (optional)

Instructions:

1. In a large pot or Dutch oven, heat the olive oil over medium heat. Add the diced onion and sauté for 5•7 minutes, until softened.

2. Add the minced garlic to the pot and cook for 1 minute, until fragrant.

3. Stir in the chopped broccoli florets, white beans, vegetable or chicken broth, dried thyme, salt, and black pepper.

4. Bring the soup to a boil, then reduce the heat and let it simmer for 15•20 minutes, or until the broccoli is tender.

5. Using an immersion blender or a regular blender, puree about half of the soup until smooth. This will help create a creamy texture.

6. Return the pureed soup to the pot and stir to combine.

7. Taste the soup and adjust the seasoning with additional salt and pepper, if desired.

8. Serve the Broccoli and White Bean Soup hot, garnished with grated Parmesan cheese if desired.

Tips:
- For a heartier meal, you can add cooked diced chicken or crumbled bacon to the soup.
- Serve the soup with crusty bread or a side salad for a complete and satisfying meal

74. Baked Cod with Herbed Quinoa

Ingredient:

Herbed Quinoa:
• 1 cup uncooked quinoa, rinsed
• 2 cups low•sodium vegetable or chicken broth
• 2 tbsp chopped fresh parsley
• 2 tbsp chopped fresh basil
• 1 tbsp chopped fresh thyme
• 1 tbsp lemon juice
• 1/4 tsp salt

Baked Cod:
• 4 (6 oz) cod fillets
• 2 tbsp olive oil
• 1 tsp paprika
• 1/2 tsp garlic powder
• 1/4 tsp salt
• 1/4 tsp black pepper

Instructions:

For the Herbed Quinoa:

1. In a medium saucepan, combine the rinsed quinoa and broth. Bring to a boil, then reduce heat to low, cover, and simmer for 15•20 minutes, or until the quinoa is tender and the liquid is absorbed.

2. Fluff the cooked quinoa with a fork and stir in the chopped parsley, basil, thyme, lemon juice, and salt. Set aside.

For the Baked Cod:

1. Preheat your oven to 400°F (200°C).

2. Place the cod fillets on a baking sheet lined with parchment paper or a silicone baking mat.

3. Drizzle the cod with the olive oil and sprinkle with the paprika, garlic powder, salt, and black pepper.

4. Bake the cod for 12•15 minutes, or until it flakes easily with a fork and is opaque throughout.

To Serve:
1. Divide the herbed quinoa among plates or bowls.

2. Top the quinoa with the baked cod fillets.

3. Serve the Baked Cod with Herbed Quinoa immediately.

Enjoy this healthy and flavorful seafood and grain dish!

75. Spinach and Mushroom Stuffed Chicken Breast

Ingredient:

- 4 boneless, skinless chicken breasts
- 8 oz fresh spinach, chopped
- 8 oz sliced mushrooms
- 2 cloves garlic, minced
- 1/4 cup grated Parmesan cheese
- 2 tbsp cream cheese, softened
- 1 tsp dried thyme
- 1/2 tsp salt
- 1/4 tsp black pepper
- 1 tbsp olive oil

Instructions:

1. Preheat your oven to 400°F (200°C).

2. In a large skillet, heat the olive oil over medium heat. Add the sliced mushrooms and sauté for 5•7 minutes, until they start to release their moisture.

3. Add the chopped spinach and minced garlic to the skillet. Cook for 2•3 minutes, stirring frequently, until the spinach is wilted. Remove from heat and let cool slightly.

4. In a medium bowl, combine the sautéed spinach and mushrooms, Parmesan cheese, cream cheese, dried thyme, salt, and black pepper. Mix well.

5. Using a sharp knife, slice a pocket into the side of each chicken breast, being careful not to cut all the way through.

6. Stuff the spinach and mushroom mixture evenly into the pockets of the chicken breasts.

7. Place the stuffed chicken breasts in a baking dish or on a rimmed baking sheet.

8. Bake the stuffed chicken breasts for 25•30 minutes, or until the chicken is cooked through and the internal temperature reaches 165°F (75°C).

9. Remove the stuffed chicken from the oven and let it rest for a few minutes before serving.

Serve the Spinach and Mushroom Stuffed Chicken Breast warm. Enjoy this delicious and healthy chicken dish!

76. Asian Slaw with Peanut Dressing

Ingredient:

Slaw:
• 2 cups shredded green cabbage
• 2 cups shredded red cabbage
• 1 cup shredded carrots
• 1/2 cup thinly sliced red onion
• 1/4 cup chopped fresh cilantro

Toppings (optional):
• 1/4 cup chopped roasted peanuts
• 2 tbsp toasted sesame seeds

Peanut Dressing:
• 1/4 cup creamy peanut butter
• 2 tbsp rice vinegar
• 2 tbsp low•sodium soy sauce
• 1 tbsp honey
• 1 tbsp sesame oil
• 1 tsp grated fresh ginger
• 1 clove garlic, minced
• 2•3 tbsp water, as needed to thin the dressing

Instructions:

1. In a large bowl, combine the shredded green cabbage, red cabbage, carrots, red onion, and chopped cilantro. Set aside.

For the Peanut Dressing:

1. In a small bowl, whisk together the peanut butter, rice vinegar, soy sauce, honey, sesame oil, grated ginger, and minced garlic.

2. Add 2•3 tablespoons of water, as needed, to thin the dressing to your desired consistency.

To Assemble:

1. Pour the peanut dressing over the slaw mixture and toss to coat the vegetables evenly.

2. Sprinkle the chopped roasted peanuts and toasted sesame seeds over the top, if using.

3. Serve the Asian Slaw with Peanut Dressing immediately or refrigerate until ready to serve.

Tips:

• For a heartier meal, you can add grilled chicken, shrimp, or tofu to the slaw.

• Customize the vegetables to your liking, such as adding shredded red bell pepper or snow peas.

• The slaw can be made in advance and the dressing can be stored separately until ready to serve.

77. Quinoa and Black Bean Stuffed Bell Peppers

Ingredient:

• 4 bell peppers (any color), halved lengthwise and seeds removed
• 1 cup cooked quinoa
• 1 (15 oz) can black beans, drained and rinsed
• 1 cup diced tomatoes
• 1/2 cup corn kernels (fresh or frozen)
• 1/4 cup chopped fresh cilantro
• 2 cloves garlic, minced
• 1 tsp ground cumin
• 1/2 tsp chili powder
• 1/4 tsp salt
• 1/4 tsp black pepper
• 1 cup shredded cheddar or Monterey Jack cheese

Instructions:

1. Preheat your oven to 375°F (190°C).

2. Arrange the bell pepper halves in a baking dish or on a rimmed baking sheet.

3. In a large bowl, combine the cooked quinoa, black beans, diced tomatoes, corn, chopped cilantro, minced garlic, ground cumin, chili powder, salt, and black pepper. Stir to mix well.

4. Spoon the quinoa and black bean mixture evenly into the bell pepper halves, pressing it down gently.

5. Top each stuffed pepper with shredded cheese.

6. Bake the stuffed peppers in the preheated oven for 25•30 minutes, or until the peppers are tender and the cheese is melted and bubbly.

7. Serve the Quinoa and Black Bean Stuffed Bell Peppers warm.

Tips:
• For extra flavor, you can add diced onion or jalapeño to the quinoa and black bean mixture.
• Serve the stuffed peppers with a side of avocado, sour cream, or salsa for a complete meal.
• This recipe can be easily doubled or tripled to serve more people.

78. Cucumber and Avocado Gazpacho

Ingredient:

• 2 cups diced cucumber
• 1 ripe avocado, pitted and diced
• 1 cup diced tomatoes
• 1/2 cup diced red onion
• 2 cloves garlic, minced
• 1/4 cup fresh cilantro, chopped
• 2 tbsp lime juice
• 1 tbsp olive oil
• 1 tsp honey
• 1/4 tsp salt
• 1/4 tsp black pepper
• 1 cup cold water or vegetable broth

Garnishes (optional):
• Diced cucumber
• Diced avocado
• Chopped cilantro
• Crumbled feta cheese

Instructions:

1. In a large bowl, combine the diced cucumber, avocado, tomatoes, red onion, garlic, cilantro, lime juice, olive oil, honey, salt, and black pepper. Stir to mix well.

2. Add the cold water or vegetable broth and stir to combine.

3. Using an immersion blender or a regular blender, puree the gazpacho mixture until smooth and creamy, leaving some small chunks for texture.

4. Taste the gazpacho and adjust the seasoning with additional salt, pepper, or lime juice if desired.

5. Cover and refrigerate the gazpacho for at least 30 minutes to allow the flavors to meld. Serve the chilled Cucumber and Avocado Gazpacho in bowls or glasses, garnished with diced cucumber, avocado, chopped cilantro, and crumbled feta cheese (if using).

Tips:
• For a thicker consistency, use less water or broth.
• You can also add a splash of white wine vinegar or sherry vinegar for extra tang.
• Garnish with toasted pumpkin seeds or crushed tortilla chips for added crunch.

79. Caprese Stuffed Portobello Mushrooms

Ingredient:

- 4 large portobello mushroom caps, stems removed
- 2 tbsp olive oil
- 1/4 tsp salt
- 1/4 tsp black pepper
- 1 cup cherry tomatoes, halved
- 1 cup fresh mozzarella cheese, diced
- 1/4 cup fresh basil leaves, chopped
- 2 tbsp balsamic glaze (or reduced balsamic vinegar)

Instructions:

1. Preheat your oven to 400°F (200°C).

2. Gently wipe the portobello mushroom caps with a damp paper towel to clean them. Remove the stems and discard or save for another use.

3. Arrange the mushroom caps, gill•side up, on a baking sheet. Drizzle the caps with the olive oil and sprinkle with salt and black pepper.

4. Bake the mushrooms for 10•12 minutes, or until they are tender and have released some of their moisture.

5. Remove the mushrooms from the oven and let them cool slightly.

6. In a medium bowl, combine the halved cherry tomatoes, diced mozzarella cheese, and chopped fresh basil. Stir to mix well.

7. Spoon the tomato•mozzarella mixture evenly into the baked mushroom caps, pressing it down gently.

8. Return the stuffed mushrooms to the oven and bake for an additional 8•10 minutes, or until the cheese is melted and bubbly.

9. Drizzle the balsamic glaze over the top of the stuffed mushrooms just before serving.

10. Serve the Caprese Stuffed Portobello Mushrooms warm.

80. Turkey and Sweet Potato Hash

Ingredient:

• 1 lb ground turkey
• 2 medium sweet potatoes, peeled and diced
• 1 red bell pepper, diced
• 1 onion, diced
• 2 cloves garlic, minced
• 1 tsp ground cumin
• 1 tsp paprika
• 1/2 tsp dried oregano
• 1/4 tsp cayenne pepper (optional)
• Salt and black pepper to taste
• 2 tbsp olive oil
• 2 cups baby spinach, chopped
• 2 tbsp chopped fresh parsley

Instructions:

1. In a large skillet or cast•iron pan, heat the olive oil over medium•high heat.

2. Add the ground turkey and cook, breaking it up with a wooden spoon, until browned and cooked through, about 5•7 minutes. Transfer the cooked turkey to a plate and set aside.

3. Add the diced sweet potatoes, bell pepper, and onion to the same skillet. Cook, stirring occasionally, until the vegetables are tender and starting to brown, about 10•12 minutes.

4. Stir in the minced garlic, ground cumin, paprika, dried oregano, and cayenne pepper (if using). Cook for 1•2 minutes, until fragrant.

5. Return the cooked turkey to the skillet and stir to combine with the vegetables. Season with salt and black pepper to taste.

6. Add the chopped baby spinach and stir until it's just wilted, about 1•2 minutes. Remove the skillet from heat and stir in the chopped fresh parsley. Serve the Turkey and Sweet Potato Hash warm.

Why this recipe supports a healthy gut and may contribute to a flat stomach:
• Sweet potatoes are a good source of fiber, which supports gut health and can help with digestion.
• Ground turkey is a lean protein that is easy to digest and can help with weight management.

81. Roasted Cauliflower and Chickpea Salad

Ingredient:

- 1 head of cauliflower, cut into florets
- 1 (15 oz) can chickpeas, drained and rinsed
- 2 tbsp olive oil
- 1 tsp ground cumin
- 1/2 tsp paprika
- 1/4 tsp cayenne pepper (optional)
- Salt and black pepper to taste
- 4 cups mixed greens (such as spinach, arugula, or kale)
- 1/4 cup crumbled feta cheese
- 2 tbsp chopped fresh parsley
- 2 tbsp lemon juice
- 1 tbsp Dijon mustard
- 1 tbsp honey

Instructions:

1. Preheat your oven to 400°F (200°C).

2. In a large bowl, toss the cauliflower florets and drained chickpeas with the olive oil, ground cumin, paprika, and cayenne pepper (if using). Season with salt and black pepper to taste.

3. Spread the seasoned cauliflower and chickpeas in a single layer on a baking sheet lined with parchment paper.

4. Roast the vegetables in the preheated oven for 20•25 minutes, stirring halfway, until the cauliflower is tender and lightly browned.

5. Remove the roasted cauliflower and chickpeas from the oven and let them cool slightly.

6. In a large salad bowl, combine the mixed greens, roasted cauliflower and chickpeas, crumbled feta cheese, and chopped fresh parsley.

7. In a small bowl, whisk together the lemon juice, Dijon mustard, and honey to make the dressing. Drizzle the dressing over the salad and toss gently to coat the ingredients evenly. Serve the Roasted Cauliflower and Chickpea Salad immediately.

82. Baked Chicken with Brussels Sprouts

Ingredient:

• 4 boneless, skinless chicken breasts
• 1 lb Brussels sprouts, trimmed and halved
• 2 tbsp olive oil
• 2 tsp dried thyme
• 1 tsp garlic powder
• 1/2 tsp salt
• 1/4 tsp black pepper
• 1/4 cup grated Parmesan cheese (optional)

Instructions:

1. Preheat your oven to 400°F (200°C).

2. In a large bowl, combine the trimmed and halved Brussels sprouts, 1 tbsp of the olive oil, 1 tsp of the dried thyme, 1/2 tsp of the garlic powder, 1/4 tsp of the salt, and 1/8 tsp of the black pepper. Toss to coat the Brussels sprouts evenly.

3. Spread the seasoned Brussels sprouts in a single layer on a large baking sheet.

4. In the same bowl, combine the chicken breasts, the remaining 1 tbsp of olive oil, 1 tsp of dried thyme, 1/2 tsp of garlic powder, 1/4 tsp of salt, and 1/8 tsp of black pepper. Rub the seasoning all over the chicken.

5. Place the seasoned chicken breasts on the baking sheet with the Brussels sprouts, making sure they are not touching each other.

6. Bake the chicken and Brussels sprouts in the preheated oven for 25•30 minutes, or until the chicken is cooked through and the Brussels sprouts are tender and lightly browned.

7. Remove the baking sheet from the oven and sprinkle the Parmesan cheese over the Brussels sprouts, if using.

8. Serve the Baked Chicken with Brussels Sprouts immediately.

This dish is a great source of protein, fiber, and nutrients that can support a healthy gut and may contribute to a flatter stomach. The Brussels sprouts are a cruciferous vegetable that is high in fiber and antioxidants, while the baked chicken provides lean protein.

83. Mango and Black Bean Quinoa Salad

Ingredient:

- 1 cup uncooked quinoa, rinsed
- 1 (15 oz) can black beans, drained and rinsed
- 1 ripe mango, diced
- 1 red bell pepper, diced
- 1/2 red onion, finely chopped
- 1/4 cup chopped fresh cilantro
- 2 tbsp lime juice
- 1 tbsp olive oil
- 1 tsp ground cumin
- 1/4 tsp salt
- 1/4 tsp black pepper

Instructions:

1. Cook the quinoa according to package instructions. Fluff with a fork and let cool.

2. In a large bowl, combine the cooked quinoa, black beans, diced mango, diced red bell pepper, chopped red onion, and chopped fresh cilantro.

3. In a small bowl, whisk together the lime juice, olive oil, ground cumin, salt, and black pepper to make the dressing.

4. Pour the dressing over the quinoa salad and toss gently to coat the ingredients evenly.

5. Refrigerate the Mango and Black Bean Quinoa Salad for at least 30 minutes to allow the flavors to meld. Serve the salad chilled or at room temperature.

This Mango and Black Bean Quinoa Salad is a great option for a healthy and gut•friendly meal. The quinoa provides a source of fiber and protein, while the black beans and mango add additional fiber, vitamins, and antioxidants. The combination of ingredients can help support a healthy gut and may contribute to a flatter stomach.

Tips:
- For extra crunch, you can add toasted slivered almonds or pepitas (pumpkin seeds) to the salad.
- Adjust the amount of lime juice, salt, and pepper to suit your taste preferences.
- This salad can be made in advance and stored in the refrigerator for up to 3•4 days.

84. Grilled Vegetable Platter with Quinoa

Ingredient:

- 2 tbsp olive oil
- 1 tsp dried oregano
- 1/2 tsp garlic powder
- 1/4 tsp salt
- 1/4 tsp black pepper
- 2 tbsp balsamic glaze (optional)
- 2 tbsp chopped fresh parsley

- 1 cup uncooked quinoa, rinsed
- 2 cups low•sodium vegetable or chicken broth
- 1 zucchini, sliced into 1/2•inch thick rounds
- 1 yellow squash, sliced into 1/2•inch thick rounds
- 1 red bell pepper, cut into 1•inch pieces
- 1 red onion, sliced into 1/2•inch thick rounds
- 8 oz cremini or button mushrooms, halved

Instructions:

1. In a medium saucepan, combine the rinsed quinoa and broth. Bring to a boil, then reduce heat to low, cover, and simmer for 15•20 minutes, or until the quinoa is tender and the liquid is absorbed. Fluff with a fork and set aside.

2. Preheat your grill or grill pan to medium•high heat.

3. In a large bowl, toss the sliced zucchini, yellow squash, bell pepper, onion, and mushrooms with the olive oil, dried oregano, garlic powder, salt, and black pepper.

4. Grill the vegetables in batches, turning occasionally, until they are tender and lightly charred, about 5•7 minutes per batch.

5. Arrange the grilled vegetables on a platter or serving dish. Top with the cooked quinoa.

6. Drizzle the balsamic glaze over the vegetables and quinoa, if using. Sprinkle the chopped fresh parsley over the top. Serve the Grilled Vegetable Platter with Quinoa warm or at room temperature.

This dish is a great source of fiber, antioxidants, and nutrients that can support a healthy gut and may contribute to a flatter stomach. The grilled vegetables provide a variety of fiber•rich and low•calorie options, while the quinoa adds protein and additional fiber. The combination of ingredients can help promote a healthy gut microbiome and aid in digestion.

85. Asian Chicken Lettuce Wraps

Ingredient:

- 1 lb ground chicken or turkey
- 2 tbsp sesame oil
- 2 tbsp low•sodium soy sauce
- 1 tbsp rice vinegar
- 1 tbsp honey
- 1 tsp grated fresh ginger
- 2 cloves garlic, minced
- 1/4 tsp red pepper flakes (optional)
- 1 cup shredded carrots
- 1 cup thinly sliced cabbage
- 1/4 cup chopped green onions
- 1/4 cup chopped fresh cilantro
- 12•16 large lettuce leaves (such as romaine, bibb, or butter lettuce)

Instructions:

1. In a large skillet or wok, cook the ground chicken or turkey over medium•high heat, breaking it up with a wooden spoon, until browned and cooked through, about 5•7 minutes. Drain any excess fat.

2. In a small bowl, whisk together the sesame oil, soy sauce, rice vinegar, honey, grated ginger, and minced garlic. Pour the sauce over the cooked chicken and stir to coat.

3. Stir in the shredded carrots, sliced cabbage, chopped green onions, and chopped cilantro. Cook for an additional 2•3 minutes, until the vegetables are slightly softened.

4. To serve, spoon the chicken and vegetable mixture into the lettuce leaves. You can serve the wraps with additional chopped green onions, cilantro, and a drizzle of the sauce, if desired.

These Asian Chicken Lettuce Wraps are a great option for a healthy and gut•friendly meal. The ground chicken or turkey provides a lean protein source, while the vegetables and lettuce leaves add fiber and nutrients that can support a healthy gut. The Asian•inspired flavors from the soy sauce, ginger, and rice vinegar can also contribute to a flatter stomach by aiding in digestion.

Enjoy these delicious and nutritious Asian Chicken Lettuce Wraps!

86. Beet and Goat Cheese Quinoa Risotto

Ingredient:

• 1 cup uncooked quinoa, rinsed
• 3 cups low•sodium vegetable or chicken broth
• 2 medium beets, peeled and diced
• 1 tbsp olive oil
• 1 shallot, minced
• 2 cloves garlic, minced
• 1/2 cup dry white wine (or additional broth)
• 4 oz crumbled goat cheese
• 2 tbsp chopped fresh parsley
• Salt and black pepper to taste

Instructions:

1. In a medium saucepan, combine the rinsed quinoa and broth. Bring to a boil, then reduce heat to low, cover, and simmer for 15•20 minutes, or until the quinoa is tender and the liquid is absorbed. Set aside.

2. In a separate saucepan, bring a small amount of water to a boil. Add the diced beets and cook for 5•7 minutes, until tender. Drain the beets and set aside.

3. In a large skillet or Dutch oven, heat the olive oil over medium heat. Add the minced shallot and garlic, and sauté for 2•3 minutes, until fragrant.

4. Add the cooked quinoa to the skillet and stir to combine with the shallot and garlic. Pour in the white wine (or additional broth) and continue to cook, stirring frequently, until the liquid is absorbed, about 5 minutes.

5. Stir in the cooked diced beets and crumbled goat cheese. Cook for an additional 2•3 minutes, until the cheese is melted and the mixture is creamy.

6. Remove the Beet and Goat Cheese Quinoa Risotto from heat and stir in the chopped fresh parsley. Season with salt and black pepper to taste. Serve the risotto warm, garnished with additional parsley if desired.

This Beet and Goat Cheese Quinoa Risotto is a great option for supporting a healthy gut and potentially contributing to a flatter stomach. The quinoa provides a source of fiber and protein, while the beets are rich in fiber, antioxidants, and nutrients that can aid digestion. The goat cheese adds a creamy texture and a boost of probiotics, which can further support gut health.

87. Shrimp and Quinoa Stuffed Bell Peppers

Ingredient:

- 4 bell peppers, halved lengthwise and seeds removed
- 1 cup cooked quinoa
- 1 lb cooked shrimp, peeled and chopped
- 1 cup diced tomatoes
- 1/2 cup diced onion
- 2 cloves garlic, minced
- 1 tsp dried oregano
- 1/2 tsp ground cumin
- 1/4 tsp red pepper flakes (optional)
- Salt and black pepper to taste
- 1/2 cup shredded mozzarella cheese

Instructions:

1. Preheat your oven to 375°F (190°C).

2. Arrange the bell pepper halves in a baking dish or on a rimmed baking sheet.

3. In a large bowl, combine the cooked quinoa, chopped shrimp, diced tomatoes, diced onion, minced garlic, dried oregano, ground cumin, and red pepper flakes (if using). Season with salt and black pepper to taste.

4. Spoon the shrimp and quinoa mixture evenly into the bell pepper halves, pressing it down gently.

5. Top each stuffed pepper with shredded mozzarella cheese.

6. Bake the stuffed peppers in the preheated oven for 25•30 minutes, or until the peppers are tender and the cheese is melted and bubbly.

7. Serve the Shrimp and Quinoa Stuffed Bell Peppers warm.

This dish is a great option for supporting a healthy gut and potentially contributing to a flatter stomach. The quinoa provides a source of fiber and protein, while the shrimp adds lean protein and beneficial omega•3 fatty acids. The bell peppers are a good source of fiber, vitamins, and antioxidants that can aid digestion and promote overall gut health.

Enjoy these delicious and nutritious Shrimp and Quinoa Stuffed Bell Peppers!

88. Greek Chicken Souvlaki with Tzatziki Sauce

Ingredient:

Tzatziki Sauce:
• 1 cup plain Greek yogurt
• 1 cucumber, peeled, seeded, and grated
• 1 clove garlic, minced
• 1 tbsp lemon juice
• 1 tbsp chopped fresh dill
• 1/4 tsp salt

To Serve:
• 8•10 wooden or metal skewers
• Pita bread or lettuce leaves
• Diced tomatoes, sliced red onion,
and crumbled feta cheese (optional)

Chicken Souvlaki:
• 1 lb boneless, skinless
chicken breasts, cut into
1•inch cubes
• 2 tbsp olive oil
• 2 tbsp lemon juice
• 1 tbsp dried oregano
• 2 cloves garlic, minced
• 1/2 tsp salt
• 1/4 tsp black pepper

Instructions:

For the Chicken Souvlaki:
1. In a large bowl, combine the cubed chicken, olive oil, lemon juice, dried oregano, minced garlic, salt, and black pepper. Toss to coat the chicken evenly.
2. Thread the marinated chicken cubes onto the skewers.

For the Tzatziki Sauce:
1. In a medium bowl, mix together the Greek yogurt, grated cucumber, minced garlic, lemon juice, chopped dill, and salt.

To Assemble:
1. Grill or broil the chicken souvlaki skewers for 8•10 minutes, turning occasionally, until the chicken is cooked through.
2. Serve the grilled chicken souvlaki skewers with the tzatziki sauce, pita bread or lettuce leaves, and any desired toppings like diced tomatoes, sliced red onion, and crumbled feta cheese.

This Greek Chicken Souvlaki with Tzatziki Sauce is a great option for supporting a healthy gut and potentially contributing to a flatter stomach. The chicken provides a lean protein source, while the tzatziki sauce is made with Greek yogurt, which contains probiotics that can aid digestion. The fresh vegetables and herbs also add fiber and nutrients that can support overall gut health.

Enjoy your delicious and healthy Greek Chicken Souvlaki with Tzatziki Sauce!

89. Spinach and Feta Turkey Burgers

Ingredient:

- 1 lb ground turkey
- 1 cup chopped fresh spinach
- 1/2 cup crumbled feta cheese
- 2 cloves garlic, minced
- 1 tsp dried oregano
- 1/2 tsp salt
- 1/4 tsp black pepper
- 4 whole wheat burger buns
- Toppings (such as tomato slices, red onion, lettuce, etc.)

Instructions:

1. In a large bowl, combine the ground turkey, chopped spinach, crumbled feta cheese, minced garlic, dried oregano, salt, and black pepper. Mix well until all the ingredients are evenly distributed.

2. Divide the turkey mixture into 4 equal portions and shape them into patties, about 4•5 inches wide and 1/2 inch thick.

3. Preheat your grill or a large skillet over medium•high heat.

4. If grilling, lightly oil the grill grates. If using a skillet, add a small amount of oil to the pan.

5. Cook the turkey burgers for 4•5 minutes per side, or until they are cooked through and reach an internal temperature of 165°F (75°C).

6. Toast the whole wheat burger buns while the burgers are cooking.

7. Place the cooked turkey burgers on the toasted buns and top with your desired toppings, such as tomato slices, red onion, and lettuce.

These Spinach and Feta Turkey Burgers are a great option for supporting a healthy gut and potentially contributing to a flatter stomach. The ground turkey provides a lean protein source, while the spinach and feta cheese add fiber, vitamins, and probiotics that can aid digestion. The whole wheat buns also contribute to the overall fiber content of the meal.

Enjoy your delicious and nutritious Spinach and Feta Turkey Burgers!

90. Coconut Curry Chicken with Brown Rice

Ingredient:

• 1 lb boneless, skinless chicken breasts, cut into 1•inch pieces
• 1 tbsp coconut oil
• 1 onion, diced
• 3 cloves garlic, minced
• 1 tbsp grated fresh ginger
• 2 tsp curry powder
• 1 tsp ground cumin
• 1/4 tsp cayenne pepper (or more to taste)
• 1 (13.5 oz) can coconut milk
• 1 cup low•sodium chicken broth
• 1 cup brown rice, cooked according to package instructions
• Chopped cilantro for serving

Instructions:

1. In a large skillet, heat the coconut oil over medium•high heat. Add the chicken and cook for 3•4 minutes until lightly browned. Remove chicken from skillet and set aside.

2. In the same skillet, add the onion and sauté for 3•4 minutes until translucent. Add the garlic and ginger and cook for 1 minute until fragrant.

3. Stir in the curry powder, cumin, and cayenne. Cook for 1 minute.

4. Pour in the coconut milk and chicken broth. Bring to a simmer and let cook for 5 minutes.

5. Add the cooked chicken back to the skillet and let simmer for 10•15 minutes until chicken is cooked through and sauce has thickened slightly.

6. Serve the coconut curry chicken over the cooked brown rice. Garnish with chopped cilantro.

Enjoy your flavorful and healthy coconut curry chicken with brown rice!

91. Tomato Basil Mozzarella Salad

Ingredient:

- 1 lb cherry or grape tomatoes, halved
- 8 oz fresh mozzarella cheese, cut into 1•inch cubes
- 1/4 cup fresh basil leaves, chopped
- 2 tbsp olive oil
- 1 tbsp balsamic vinegar
- 1 tsp Dijon mustard
- 1 garlic clove, minced
- Salt and pepper to taste

Instructions:

1. In a large bowl, combine the halved tomatoes, mozzarella cubes, and chopped basil.

2. In a small bowl, whisk together the olive oil, balsamic vinegar, Dijon mustard, and minced garlic. Season with salt and pepper to taste.

3. Pour the dressing over the tomato, mozzarella, and basil mixture and gently toss to coat everything evenly.

4. Let the salad sit for 5•10 minutes to allow the flavors to meld together.

5. Serve immediately or chill in the refrigerator until ready to serve.

This fresh and flavorful Tomato Basil Mozzarella Salad makes a great side dish or light main course. The combination of juicy tomatoes, creamy mozzarella, and fragrant basil is simply delicious. Adjust the amounts of each ingredient to your taste preferences.

Enjoy!

92. Baked Tofu with Stir•fried Vegetables

Ingredient:

For the Baked Tofu:
• 1 block (14 oz) extra•firm tofu, pressed and cut into 1•inch cubes
• 2 tbsp soy sauce
• 1 tbsp sesame oil
• 1 tbsp cornstarch

For the Stir•Fried Vegetables:
• 2 tbsp sesame oil
• 3 cloves garlic, minced
• 1 inch fresh ginger, peeled and grated
• 1 red bell pepper, sliced
• 1 cup broccoli florets
• 1 cup snow peas or snap peas
• 2 cups baby spinach
• 2 tbsp soy sauce
• 1 tbsp rice vinegar
• Salt and pepper to taste
• Cooked brown rice, for serving

Instructions:
1. Preheat the oven to 400°F. Line a baking sheet with parchment paper.

For the Baked Tofu:
2. In a bowl, toss the tofu cubes with the soy sauce, sesame oil, and cornstarch until evenly coated.
3. Arrange the tofu cubes in a single layer on the prepared baking sheet. Bake for 20•25 minutes, flipping halfway, until golden brown.

For the Stir•Fried Vegetables:
4. In a large skillet or wok, heat the sesame oil over medium•high heat. Add the garlic and ginger and cook for 1 minute until fragrant.
5. Add the bell pepper, broccoli, and snow peas. Stir•fry for 3•4 minutes until vegetables are crisp•tender.
6. Add the spinach and stir•fry for 1 minute until wilted.
7. Stir in the soy sauce and rice vinegar. Season with salt and pepper to taste.

To Serve:
8. Serve the baked tofu and stir•fried vegetables over cooked brown rice.

93. Green Goddess Salad with Chicken

Ingredient:

For the Salad:
• 6 cups mixed greens (such as romaine, spinach, and arugula)
• 1 cup cooked chicken breast, shredded or diced
• 1 avocado, diced
• 1 cup cucumber, diced
• 1/2 cup cherry tomatoes, halved
• 1/4 cup crumbled feta cheese
• 2 tbsp toasted sunflower seeds

For the Green Goddess Dressing:
• 1/2 cup plain Greek yogurt
• 1/4 cup fresh parsley
• 2 tbsp fresh chives, chopped
• 1 tbsp fresh tarragon, chopped
• 1 tbsp lemon juice
• 1 garlic clove, minced
• 1 tsp Dijon mustard
• 1/4 tsp salt
• 1/8 tsp black pepper

Instructions:

1. Make the Green Goddess Dressing: In a food processor or blender, combine all the dressing ingredients and blend until smooth and creamy. Taste and adjust seasoning as needed.

2. In a large salad bowl, combine the mixed greens, cooked chicken, avocado, cucumber, cherry tomatoes, feta cheese, and sunflower seeds.

3. Drizzle the Green Goddess Dressing over the salad and gently toss to coat everything evenly.

4. Serve the Green Goddess Salad immediately.

This fresh and flavorful Green Goddess Salad with Chicken makes a delicious and nutritious meal. The creamy, herb•infused dressing pairs perfectly with the crunchy vegetables, juicy chicken, and creamy avocado. Feel free to adjust the ingredient amounts to your taste preferences.

94. Cauliflower Rice Sushi Rolls

Ingredient:

• 1 head of cauliflower, riced
• 2 tbsp rice vinegar
• 1 tsp sugar
• 1/4 tsp salt
• 4•6 sheets of nori (seaweed sheets)
• Fillings of your choice (e.g. avocado, cucumber, carrots, cooked shrimp, crab meat)
• Soy sauce, for serving

Instructions:

1. Make the cauliflower rice: Pulse the cauliflower florets in a food processor until they resemble rice•sized grains. Transfer the cauliflower rice to a microwave•safe bowl and microwave for 2•3 minutes until softened.

2. In a small bowl, mix together the rice vinegar, sugar, and salt. Pour this mixture over the warm cauliflower rice and stir to combine. Allow the cauliflower rice to cool slightly.

3. Lay a sheet of nori on a sushi mat or clean, flat surface. Spread about 1/2 cup of the cauliflower rice in an even layer over the nori, leaving about 1 inch of nori uncovered at the top.

4. Arrange your desired fillings in a line across the center of the cauliflower rice.

5. Using the sushi mat, carefully roll the nori and fillings up tightly, starting from the bottom and rolling towards the uncovered top edge. Moisten the uncovered edge with a bit of water to help seal the roll.

6. Slice the sushi roll into 6•8 pieces using a sharp knife. Repeat with remaining nori sheets and fillings.

7. Serve the cauliflower rice sushi rolls with soy sauce for dipping.

Enjoy these low•carb, veggie•packed sushi rolls! Feel free to get creative with different fillings.

95. Lemon Garlic Shrimp with Quinoa

Ingredient:

- 1 cup uncooked quinoa, rinsed
- 2 cups low•sodium chicken or vegetable broth
- 1 lb large shrimp, peeled and deveined
- 2 tbsp olive oil
- 3 cloves garlic, minced
- 1 tsp lemon zest
- 2 tbsp lemon juice
- 1/4 tsp red pepper flakes (optional)
- 2 tbsp chopped fresh parsley
- Salt and pepper to taste

Instructions:

1. In a medium saucepan, combine the quinoa and broth. Bring to a boil, then reduce heat to low, cover and simmer for 15•20 minutes until quinoa is tender and liquid is absorbed. Fluff with a fork.

2. In a large skillet, heat the olive oil over medium•high heat. Add the garlic and cook for 1 minute until fragrant.

3. Add the shrimp to the skillet and cook for 2•3 minutes per side, until the shrimp are opaque and cooked through.

4. Stir in the lemon zest, lemon juice, and red pepper flakes (if using). Season with salt and pepper to taste.

5. Remove the skillet from heat and stir in the chopped parsley.

6. To serve, divide the cooked quinoa among plates and top with the lemon garlic shrimp.

This Lemon Garlic Shrimp with Quinoa makes a light, healthy, and flavorful meal. The bright lemon and garlic flavors pair perfectly with the tender shrimp and nutty quinoa. Adjust the amount of red pepper flakes to your desired spice level.

Enjoy!

96. Turkey and Spinach Meatballs

Ingredient:

- 1 lb ground turkey
- 1 cup fresh spinach, finely chopped
- 1/2 cup breadcrumbs
- 1/4 cup grated Parmesan cheese
- 1 egg
- 2 cloves garlic, minced
- 1 tsp dried oregano
- 1/2 tsp salt
- 1/4 tsp black pepper
- 2 tbsp olive oil

Instructions:

1. Preheat your oven to 400°F. Line a baking sheet with parchment paper.

2. In a large bowl, combine the ground turkey, chopped spinach, breadcrumbs, Parmesan, egg, garlic, oregano, salt, and pepper. Mix well until all the ingredients are evenly distributed.

3. Scoop out about 2 tablespoons of the turkey mixture and roll it into a ball with your hands. Place the meatball on the prepared baking sheet. Repeat with the remaining mixture to make about 20•24 meatballs.

4. Drizzle the meatballs with the olive oil, making sure to coat them evenly.

5. Bake the meatballs for 18•20 minutes, flipping them halfway through, until they are cooked through and lightly browned.

6. Serve the turkey and spinach meatballs warm, either on their own or with your favorite pasta, sauce, or vegetable side dish.

These healthy turkey and spinach meatballs are packed with flavor and nutrients. The spinach adds a nice boost of vitamins and minerals, while the Parmesan and breadcrumbs help bind the meatballs together. Enjoy!

97. Stuffed Delicata Squash with Quinoa and Kale

Ingredient:

- 2 delicata squash, halved lengthwise and seeds removed
- 1 cup cooked quinoa
- 1 cup chopped kale, stems removed
- 1/2 cup crumbled feta cheese
- 2 tbsp olive oil, divided
- 2 cloves garlic, minced
- 1 tsp dried thyme
- Salt and pepper to taste

Instructions:

1. Preheat your oven to 400°F. Line a baking sheet with parchment paper.

2. Place the delicata squash halves cut•side up on the prepared baking sheet. Drizzle with 1 tbsp of the olive oil and season with salt and pepper. Roast for 20•25 minutes, until the squash is tender when pierced with a fork.

3. While the squash is roasting, heat the remaining 1 tbsp of olive oil in a skillet over medium heat. Add the minced garlic and sauté for 1 minute until fragrant.

4. Add the chopped kale to the skillet and cook for 2•3 minutes, until the kale is wilted. Remove from heat and let cool slightly.

5. In a medium bowl, combine the cooked quinoa, sautéed kale, crumbled feta, and dried thyme. Season with salt and pepper to taste.

6. Once the squash is roasted, scoop the quinoa and kale mixture evenly into the squash halves.

7. Return the stuffed squash to the oven and bake for an additional 10•15 minutes, until the filling is heated through.

8. Serve the stuffed delicata squash warm. Enjoy!

This Stuffed Delicata Squash with Quinoa and Kale makes a delicious and nutritious vegetarian main dish or side. The sweet roasted squash pairs perfectly with the savory quinoa, kale, and feta filling.

98. Teriyaki Tofu and Broccoli Stir•fry

Ingredient:

- 1 block (14 oz) extra•firm tofu, pressed and cut into 1•inch cubes
- 2 tbsp cornstarch
- 2 tbsp vegetable oil, divided
- 3 cups broccoli florets
- 2 cloves garlic, minced
- 1 inch fresh ginger, peeled and grated
- 1/2 cup teriyaki sauce
- 2 tbsp low•sodium soy sauce
- 1 tsp sesame oil
- Cooked brown rice, for serving

Instructions:

1. In a large bowl, toss the tofu cubes with the cornstarch until evenly coated.

2. In a large skillet or wok, heat 1 tbsp of the vegetable oil over medium•high heat. Add the coated tofu cubes and cook for 3•4 minutes per side, until golden brown. Transfer the tofu to a plate and set aside.

3. In the same skillet, heat the remaining 1 tbsp of vegetable oil. Add the broccoli florets and stir•fry for 3•4 minutes until crisp•tender.

4. Add the minced garlic and grated ginger to the skillet and cook for 1 minute until fragrant.

5. Pour in the teriyaki sauce and soy sauce. Bring the mixture to a simmer and let cook for 2•3 minutes, until the sauce has thickened slightly.

6. Add the cooked tofu back to the skillet and toss everything together to coat the tofu in the sauce.

7. Remove from heat and drizzle with the sesame oil.

8. Serve the teriyaki tofu and broccoli stir•fry over cooked brown rice.

Enjoy this flavorful and healthy Teriyaki Tofu and Broccoli Stir•Fry! The crispy tofu and tender broccoli pair perfectly with the sweet and savory teriyaki sauce.

99. Butternut Squash and Kale Salad

Ingredient:

- 1 small butternut squash, peeled, seeded, and cubed (about 3 cups)
- 2 tbsp olive oil
- Salt and pepper to taste
- 4 cups chopped kale, stems removed
- 1/2 cup crumbled feta cheese
- 1/4 cup toasted pumpkin seeds
- 2 tbsp balsamic vinegar
- 1 tbsp honey
- 1 tsp Dijon mustard

Instructions:

1. Preheat your oven to 400°F. Line a baking sheet with parchment paper.

2. Toss the cubed butternut squash with 1 tbsp of the olive oil. Season with salt and pepper. Spread the squash in a single layer on the prepared baking sheet.

3. Roast the butternut squash for 20•25 minutes, stirring halfway, until tender and lightly browned. Allow to cool slightly.

4. In a large salad bowl, combine the roasted butternut squash, chopped kale, crumbled feta, and toasted pumpkin seeds.

5. In a small bowl, whisk together the remaining 1 tbsp olive oil, balsamic vinegar, honey, and Dijon mustard. Season the dressing with salt and pepper to taste.

6. Drizzle the dressing over the salad and toss gently to coat everything evenly.

7. Serve the Butternut Squash and Kale Salad immediately.

This salad is a delicious and nutritious combination of sweet roasted butternut squash, nutrient•dense kale, creamy feta, and crunchy pumpkin seeds. The balsamic vinaigrette adds a nice tangy and sweet flavor. Enjoy!

100. Mediterranean Stuffed Peppers

Ingredient:

• 4 bell peppers (any color), halved lengthwise and seeds removed
• 1 cup cooked quinoa
• 1 (15 oz) can chickpeas, drained and rinsed
• 1 cup diced tomatoes
• 1/2 cup crumbled feta cheese
• 1/4 cup chopped fresh parsley
• 2 cloves garlic, minced
• 1 tsp dried oregano
• 1/4 tsp red pepper flakes (optional)
• Salt and pepper to taste
• 2 tbsp olive oil

Instructions:

1. Preheat your oven to 375°F. Lightly grease a baking dish or line it with parchment paper.

2. Arrange the bell pepper halves cut•side up in the prepared baking dish.

3. In a large bowl, combine the cooked quinoa, chickpeas, diced tomatoes, feta cheese, parsley, garlic, oregano, and red pepper flakes (if using). Season with salt and pepper to taste.

4. Spoon the quinoa and vegetable mixture evenly into the bell pepper halves.

5. Drizzle the stuffed peppers with the olive oil.

6. Bake the stuffed peppers for 25•30 minutes, until the peppers are tender and the filling is hot.

7. Serve the Mediterranean Stuffed Peppers warm. Enjoy!

These Mediterranean Stuffed Peppers make a delicious and healthy vegetarian main dish or side. The quinoa, chickpeas, and feta provide protein and fiber, while the fresh herbs and spices add tons of flavor. Feel free to customize the filling with your favorite Mediterranean ingredients.

101. Lemon Herb Baked Cod with Quinoa

Ingredient:

- 1 cup uncooked quinoa, rinsed
- 2 cups low•sodium chicken or vegetable broth
- 1 lb cod fillets, cut into 4 portions
- 2 tbsp olive oil
- 2 tbsp lemon juice
- 2 tsp lemon zest
- 2 tbsp chopped fresh parsley
- 1 tbsp chopped fresh dill
- 2 cloves garlic, minced
- 1/4 tsp salt
- 1/4 tsp black pepper

Instructions:

1. Preheat your oven to 400°F. Lightly grease a baking dish.

2. In a medium saucepan, combine the quinoa and broth. Bring to a boil, then reduce heat to low, cover and simmer for 15•20 minutes until quinoa is tender and liquid is absorbed. Fluff with a fork.

3. In a small bowl, mix together the olive oil, lemon juice, lemon zest, parsley, dill, garlic, salt, and pepper.

4. Place the cod fillets in the prepared baking dish. Spoon the lemon herb mixture evenly over the top of the cod.

5. Bake the cod for 12•15 minutes, until it flakes easily with a fork and is opaque throughout.

6. Serve the baked lemon herb cod immediately over the cooked quinoa.

This Lemon Herb Baked Cod with Quinoa is a light, healthy, and flavorful meal. The tender, flaky cod is perfectly complemented by the bright lemon and fresh herbs. The nutty quinoa provides a nutritious base. Enjoy!

102. Chickpea and Avocado Salad

Ingredient:

- 1 (15 oz) can chickpeas, drained and rinsed
- 1 avocado, diced
- 1/2 cup cherry tomatoes, halved
- 1/4 cup diced red onion
- 2 tbsp chopped fresh cilantro
- 2 tbsp olive oil
- 1 tbsp lemon juice
- 1 tsp Dijon mustard
- 1/4 tsp salt
- 1/8 tsp black pepper

Instructions:

1. In a large bowl, combine the drained and rinsed chickpeas, diced avocado, cherry tomatoes, red onion, and chopped cilantro.

2. In a small bowl, whisk together the olive oil, lemon juice, Dijon mustard, salt, and black pepper to make the dressing.

3. Pour the dressing over the chickpea and avocado mixture and gently toss to coat everything evenly.

4. Serve the Chickpea and Avocado Salad immediately, or refrigerate for 30 minutes to allow the flavors to meld.

This Chickpea and Avocado Salad makes a delicious and nutritious lunch or side dish. The creamy avocado, protein•packed chickpeas, and fresh vegetables are tossed in a tangy lemon•Dijon dressing.

You can customize this salad by adding other ingredients like diced cucumber, crumbled feta, or chopped nuts. It's also great served on a bed of greens or with whole grain crackers or pita bread.

Enjoy this fresh and flavorful Chickpea and Avocado Salad!

103. Grilled Chicken and Vegetable Skewers

Ingredient:

- 1 lb boneless, skinless chicken breasts, cut into 1•inch cubes
- 1 red bell pepper, cut into 1•inch pieces
- 1 zucchini, cut into 1•inch pieces
- 1 red onion, cut into 1•inch pieces
- 8 oz mushrooms, halved
- 2 tbsp olive oil
- 2 tbsp lemon juice
- 2 tsp dried oregano
- 1 tsp garlic powder
- 1/2 tsp salt
- 1/4 tsp black pepper

Instructions:

1. In a large bowl, combine the cubed chicken, bell pepper, zucchini, red onion, and mushrooms.

2. In a small bowl, whisk together the olive oil, lemon juice, oregano, garlic powder, salt, and black pepper. Pour the marinade over the chicken and vegetables and toss to coat everything evenly.

3. Thread the marinated chicken and vegetables onto metal or wooden skewers, alternating the ingredients.

4. Preheat your grill or grill pan to medium•high heat.

5. Grill the skewers for 12•15 minutes, turning occasionally, until the chicken is cooked through and the vegetables are tender.

6. Serve the Grilled Chicken and Vegetable Skewers immediately.

These colorful and flavorful skewers make a great main dish or appetizer. The combination of juicy chicken, crisp vegetables, and the zesty marinade is simply delicious.

You can adjust the vegetable selection based on your preferences. Serve the skewers with a side of rice, quinoa, or a fresh salad for a complete and healthy meal.

Enjoy your Grilled Chicken and Vegetable Skewers!

104. Cilantro Lime Shrimp with Brown Rice

Ingredient:

• 1 cup uncooked brown rice
• 1 lb large shrimp, peeled and deveined
• 2 tbsp olive oil
• 3 cloves garlic, minced
• 1 tsp ground cumin
• 1/4 tsp cayenne pepper (optional)
• 1/4 cup chopped fresh cilantro
• 2 tbsp fresh lime juice
• Salt and pepper to taste

Instructions:

1. Cook the brown rice according to package instructions. Set aside.

2. In a large skillet, heat the olive oil over medium•high heat. Add the minced garlic and cook for 1 minute until fragrant.

3. Add the shrimp, cumin, and cayenne pepper (if using) to the skillet. Cook for 2•3 minutes per side, until the shrimp are opaque and cooked through.

4. Remove the skillet from heat and stir in the chopped cilantro and lime juice. Season with salt and pepper to taste.

5. To serve, divide the cooked brown rice among plates and top with the cilantro lime shrimp.

This Cilantro Lime Shrimp with Brown Rice is a quick, easy, and flavorful meal. The bright, zesty flavors of the cilantro and lime pair perfectly with the tender shrimp. The nutty brown rice provides a nutritious base.

You can adjust the amount of cayenne pepper to control the heat level. Serve with additional lime wedges, if desired.

Enjoy this healthy and delicious shrimp and rice dish!

105. Baked Stuffed Apples with Greek Yogurt

Ingredient:

- 4 medium•sized apples (such as Honeycrisp or Gala)
- 1/2 cup rolled oats
- 1/4 cup chopped walnuts
- 2 tbsp brown sugar
- 1 tsp ground cinnamon
- 1/4 tsp ground nutmeg
- 2 tbsp unsalted butter, melted
- 1 cup plain Greek yogurt, for serving

Instructions:

1. Preheat your oven to 375°F. Lightly grease a baking dish.

2. Cut the tops off the apples and use a melon baller or small spoon to scoop out the cores, leaving about 1/2 inch of the apple intact at the bottom. Place the hollowed•out apples in the prepared baking dish.

3. In a small bowl, combine the rolled oats, chopped walnuts, brown sugar, cinnamon, and nutmeg. Stir to mix well.

4. Spoon the oat mixture evenly into the hollowed•out apples. Drizzle the melted butter over the top of the stuffed apples.

5. Bake the stuffed apples for 30•35 minutes, until the apples are tender and the topping is golden brown.

6. Remove the baked stuffed apples from the oven and let them cool for 5 minutes.

7. Serve the warm baked apples with a dollop of plain Greek yogurt on top.

These Baked Stuffed Apples with Greek Yogurt make a delicious and healthy dessert or snack. The sweet, cinnamon•spiced apples are perfectly complemented by the creamy, tangy Greek yogurt. Enjoy!

106. Tuna and White Bean Salad

Ingredient:

• 1 (15 oz) can white beans, drained and rinsed
• 1 (5 oz) can tuna, drained
• 1/2 cup diced celery
• 1/4 cup diced red onion
• 2 tbsp chopped fresh parsley
• 2 tbsp olive oil
• 1 tbsp lemon juice
• 1 tsp Dijon mustard
• 1/4 tsp salt
• 1/8 tsp black pepper

Instructions:

1. In a medium bowl, gently combine the drained and rinsed white beans, drained tuna, diced celery, diced red onion, and chopped parsley.

2. In a small bowl, whisk together the olive oil, lemon juice, Dijon mustard, salt, and black pepper to make the dressing.

3. Pour the dressing over the tuna and white bean mixture and toss gently to coat everything evenly.

4. Serve the Tuna and White Bean Salad immediately, or refrigerate for 30 minutes to allow the flavors to meld.

This Tuna and White Bean Salad makes a quick, easy, and nutritious lunch or light dinner. The combination of protein•rich tuna, fiber•filled white beans, and fresh vegetables is both satisfying and delicious.

You can customize this salad by adding other ingredients like diced cucumber, cherry tomatoes, or crumbled feta cheese. It's also great served on a bed of greens or with whole grain crackers or pita bread.

Enjoy this simple and flavorful Tuna and White Bean Salad!

107. Veggie Stir•fry with Brown Rice

Ingredient:

- 1 cup uncooked brown rice
- 2 tbsp sesame oil
- 3 cloves garlic, minced
- 1 inch fresh ginger, peeled and grated
- 1 red bell pepper, sliced
- 1 cup broccoli florets
- 1 cup snow peas or snap peas
- 1 cup sliced mushrooms
- 2 cups baby spinach
- 2 tbsp low•sodium soy sauce
- 1 tbsp rice vinegar
- Salt and pepper to taste

Instructions:

1. Cook the brown rice according to package instructions. Set aside.

2. In a large skillet or wok, heat the sesame oil over medium•high heat. Add the minced garlic and grated ginger and cook for 1 minute until fragrant.

3. Add the sliced red bell pepper, broccoli florets, snow peas/snap peas, and sliced mushrooms to the skillet. Stir•fry for 4•5 minutes until the vegetables are crisp•tender.

4. Add the baby spinach to the skillet and cook for 1•2 minutes until the spinach is wilted.

5. Stir in the soy sauce and rice vinegar. Season with salt and pepper to taste.

6. Serve the veggie stir•fry immediately over the cooked brown rice.

This Veggie Stir•Fry with Brown Rice is a healthy, flavorful, and easy•to•make meal. The combination of fresh vegetables, savory soy sauce, and nutty brown rice makes for a satisfying and nutritious dish.

Feel free to substitute or add other vegetables based on your preferences. You can also adjust the amount of soy sauce and vinegar to suit your taste.

Enjoy this delicious and wholesome Veggie Stir•Fry with Brown Rice!

108. Spinach and Quinoa Stuffed Tomatoes

Ingredient:

• 6 medium tomatoes
• 1 cup cooked quinoa
• 1 cup chopped fresh spinach
• 1/4 cup crumbled feta cheese
• 2 tbsp chopped fresh basil
• 1 clove garlic, minced
• 1 tbsp olive oil
• Salt and pepper to taste

Instructions:

1. Preheat your oven to 375°F. Line a baking sheet with parchment paper.

2. Slice the tops off the tomatoes and scoop out the insides, leaving a 1/4•inch shell. Finely chop the scooped out tomato flesh.

3. In a medium bowl, combine the chopped tomato flesh, cooked quinoa, chopped spinach, crumbled feta, chopped basil, minced garlic, and olive oil. Season with salt and pepper to taste.

4. Stuff the quinoa and spinach mixture evenly into the hollowed•out tomato shells.

5. Place the stuffed tomatoes on the prepared baking sheet.

6. Bake the stuffed tomatoes for 20•25 minutes, until the tomatoes are softened and the filling is heated through.

7. Serve the Spinach and Quinoa Stuffed Tomatoes warm.

These Spinach and Quinoa Stuffed Tomatoes make a delicious and healthy vegetarian main dish or side. The juicy tomatoes are filled with a flavorful mixture of nutrient•dense quinoa, fresh spinach, and tangy feta. The basil and garlic add wonderful aromatic notes.

You can customize the filling by adding other chopped vegetables, herbs, or even cooked chickpeas or lentils. Enjoy these tasty and nutritious stuffed tomatoes!

109. Turkey and Quinoa Stuffed Acorn Squash

Ingredient:

- 2 acorn squash, halved and seeded
- 1 lb ground turkey
- 1 cup cooked quinoa
- 1 cup chopped kale
- 1/2 cup diced onion
- 2 cloves garlic, minced
- 1 tsp dried thyme
- 1/2 tsp salt
- 1/4 tsp black pepper
- 1/4 cup shredded mozzarella cheese

Instructions:

1. Preheat your oven to 400°F. Line a baking sheet with parchment paper.

2. Place the acorn squash halves cut•side down on the prepared baking sheet. Roast for 30•35 minutes, until the squash is tender when pierced with a fork.

3. In a large skillet, cook the ground turkey over medium heat, breaking it up with a wooden spoon, until no longer pink, about 5•7 minutes.

4. Add the cooked quinoa, chopped kale, diced onion, minced garlic, dried thyme, salt, and pepper to the skillet with the turkey. Stir to combine and cook for 2•3 minutes until the kale is wilted.

5. Flip the roasted acorn squash halves over so they are cut•side up. Scoop the turkey and quinoa mixture evenly into the squash cavities.

6. Sprinkle the shredded mozzarella cheese over the top of the stuffed squash.

7. Return the stuffed squash to the oven and bake for an additional 10•15 minutes, until the cheese is melted and bubbly.

8. Serve the Turkey and Quinoa Stuffed Acorn Squash warm.

This hearty and nutritious stuffed squash dish makes a delicious main course. The combination of savory turkey, nutty quinoa, and tender acorn squash is simply delicious. Enjoy!

110. Mediterranean Quinoa Salad

Ingredient:

- 1 cup uncooked quinoa, rinsed
- 2 cups vegetable or chicken broth
- 1 cup cherry tomatoes, halved
- 1 cucumber, diced
- 1 cup crumbled feta cheese
- 1/2 cup kalamata olives, sliced
- 1/4 cup chopped fresh parsley
- 2 tbsp chopped fresh basil
- 2 tbsp olive oil
- 2 tbsp lemon juice
- 1 tsp Dijon mustard
- 1 clove garlic, minced
- 1/4 tsp salt
- 1/8 tsp black pepper

Instructions:

1. In a medium saucepan, combine the rinsed quinoa and broth. Bring to a boil, then reduce heat to low, cover and simmer for 15•20 minutes until quinoa is tender and liquid is absorbed. Fluff with a fork and let cool.

2. In a large bowl, combine the cooked and cooled quinoa, cherry tomatoes, diced cucumber, crumbled feta, sliced olives, chopped parsley, and chopped basil.

3. In a small bowl, whisk together the olive oil, lemon juice, Dijon mustard, minced garlic, salt, and pepper to make the dressing.

4. Pour the dressing over the quinoa salad and toss gently to coat everything evenly.

5. Refrigerate the Mediterranean Quinoa Salad for at least 30 minutes to allow the flavors to meld.

6. Serve chilled or at room temperature.

This fresh and flavorful Mediterranean Quinoa Salad makes a great side dish or light main course. The combination of protein•rich quinoa, fresh vegetables, briny olives, and tangy feta is simply delicious. Adjust any ingredients to your taste preferences.

111. Baked Sweet Potato with Kale and Tahini Drizzle

Ingredient:

- 2 medium sweet potatoes, scrubbed clean
- 2 cups chopped kale, stems removed
- 1 tbsp olive oil
- 2 tbsp tahini
- 1 tbsp lemon juice
- 1 tbsp water
- 1 garlic clove, minced
- 1/4 tsp ground cumin
- Salt and pepper to taste

Instructions:

1. Preheat your oven to 400°F. Line a baking sheet with parchment paper.

2. Pierce the sweet potatoes a few times with a fork. Place them directly on the oven rack and bake for 45•55 minutes, until very soft when squeezed.

3. In a skillet, heat the olive oil over medium heat. Add the chopped kale and sauté for 3•4 minutes, until wilted and tender. Season with a pinch of salt and pepper.

4. In a small bowl, whisk together the tahini, lemon juice, water, minced garlic, and ground cumin. Season with salt and pepper to taste.

5. Once the sweet potatoes are cooked, slice them open lengthwise. Fluff the insides with a fork.

6. Top the baked sweet potato halves with the sautéed kale. Drizzle the tahini sauce over the top.

7. Serve the Baked Sweet Potato with Kale and Tahini Drizzle immediately.

This nutritious and flavorful dish combines the natural sweetness of baked sweet potatoes with the earthy kale and the creamy, nutty tahini sauce. It makes a delicious and satisfying vegetarian meal or side.

Feel free to adjust the amount of tahini sauce to your taste preferences. Enjoy this wholesome and delicious baked sweet potato!

112. Grilled Lemon Herb Chicken with Asparagus

Ingredient:

- 1 lb boneless, skinless chicken breasts
- 2 tbsp olive oil
- 2 tbsp lemon juice
- 2 tsp dried oregano
- 1 tsp dried thyme
- 1 tsp garlic powder
- 1/2 tsp salt
- 1/4 tsp black pepper
- 1 lb asparagus, trimmed
- Lemon wedges for serving

Instructions:

1. In a shallow dish, combine the olive oil, lemon juice, oregano, thyme, garlic powder, salt, and pepper. Add the chicken breasts and turn to coat both sides. Cover and marinate for 30 minutes to 1 hour.

2. Preheat your grill or grill pan to medium•high heat.

3. Grill the chicken for 5•7 minutes per side, until cooked through and no longer pink in the center. Transfer the grilled chicken to a plate and cover to keep warm.

4. Add the trimmed asparagus spears to the grill and cook for 3•5 minutes, turning occasionally, until tender•crisp.

5. Serve the grilled lemon herb chicken immediately, with the grilled asparagus on the side. Garnish with lemon wedges.

This Grilled Lemon Herb Chicken with Asparagus is a simple, healthy, and flavorful meal. The bright lemon and aromatic herbs complement the juicy chicken and tender asparagus perfectly.

You can adjust the cooking time for the chicken and asparagus based on their thickness. Serve with your favorite sides, such as roasted potatoes or a fresh salad.

Enjoy this delicious and easy•to•make grilled chicken and asparagus dish!

Congratulations on completing your journey through the ***"Healthy Gut Flat Stomach Cookbook: 100+ Nutritious Recipes to Support Gut Health and Achieve a Flat Stomach."*** We hope this cookbook has inspired you to embrace the power of wholesome, gut-nourishing recipes and empowered you to achieve your health and wellness goals.

Reflecting on Your Health Journey

Throughout this cookbook, you've explored over 100 delicious and nutritious recipes designed to enhance digestive wellness and support a flat stomach. By incorporating ingredients rich in fiber, probiotics, antioxidants, and essential nutrients, you've taken proactive steps towards improving digestion, reducing bloating, and achieving a toned midsection.

Celebrating Your Culinary Successes

As you reflect on the recipes you've tried and the meals you've enjoyed, take pride in your culinary accomplishments. Each dish you've prepared has not only nourished your body but also contributed to your overall well-being. Cooking is an act of self-care and creativity, and you've embraced both with every meal you've made.

Continuing Your Wellness Journey

Your journey towards digestive health and a flat stomach doesn't end here. Use the knowledge and recipes you've gained from this cookbook as a foundation to continue exploring and experimenting with gut-friendly ingredients and healthy cooking techniques. Whether you're preparing meals for yourself, your family, or friends, continue to prioritize nourishing your body with wholesome, balanced foods.

Embracing a Healthy Lifestyle

Beyond the kitchen, remember that achieving and maintaining digestive wellness and a flat stomach is a holistic journey. Incorporate regular physical activity, prioritize hydration, manage stress levels, and get adequate sleep to support your overall health goals. A balanced lifestyle complements the nutritious meals you've enjoyed from this cookbook.

Your Commitment to Well-Being

Thank you for choosing the "Healthy Gut Flat Stomach Cookbook" as your guide to better health through nutrition. By investing in your gut health and embracing these recipes, you've demonstrated a commitment to your well-being and vitality. Continue to listen to your body, make mindful food choices, and celebrate the positive impact that nutritious eating has on your life.